MCQ Companion to the Textbook of Anaesthesia

David Fell
BSc MB ChB FCAnaes
Senior Lecturer,
University of Leicester,
Leicester, UK

David R. Derbyshire
MB ChB FCAnaes
Consultant Anaesthetist,
South Warwickshire Hospital,
Warwick, UK

Alan R. Aitkenhead
BSc MD FCAnaes
Professor of Anaesthesia,
University of Nottingham,
Nottingham, UK

Graham Smith
BSc (Hons) MD FCAnaes
Professor of Anaesthesia,
University of Leicester,
Leicester, UK

Churchill Livingstone
EDINBURGH LONDON MELBOURNE NEW YORK AND TOKYO 1991

CHURCHILL LIVINGSTONE
Medical Division of Longman Group UK Limited

Distributed in the United States of America by Churchill
Livingstone Inc., 650 Avenue of the Americas, New York,
N.Y. 10011, and by associated companies, branches and
representatives throughout the world.

First published 1991
  Reprinted 1993

ISBN 0-443-04063-X

British Library Cataloguing in Publication Data
CIP catalogue record for this book is available from the
British Library.
Library of Congress Cataloging in Publication Data
CIP catalog record for this book is available from the
Library of Congress.

The
publisher's
policy is to use
**paper manufactured
from sustainable forests**

Produced by Longman Singapore Publishers (Pte) Ltd.
Printed in Singapore

Preface

This Book has been designed primarily to serve two major roles; firstly to act as a companion to the *Textbook of Anaesthesia*, 2nd edition, edited by A R Aitkenhead and G Smith, and secondly to provide examination practice at multiple choice questions (MCQ) for the FCAnaes Part 1 examination.

In its first role, we have attempted to provide cross references to a large amount of material in the *Textbook of Anaesthesia*; thus readers should be able to test themselves on how well they assimilate information and concepts at a level appropriate for the FCAnaes Part 1 examination.

The multiple choice examination question paper represents a major hurdle for many candidates undertaking higher examinations. Whilst there are already in existence several books presenting MCQs in anaesthesia and clinical practice, none is designed specifically for the Part 1 FCAnaes examination. The second major role of this book therefore represents our attempts to fill this void. The encouraging response to publication of the first edition of the *Textbook of Anaesthesia* suggested that it was useful in fulfilling one of its aims in providing suitable reading material for anaesthetists studying for the FCAnaes Part 1 examination. It should follow that an MCQ book based on the *Textbook of Anaesthesia* should also contain material appropriate to this examination and to the new recruit into anaesthesia during the first 1–2 years in the specialty. However, the examination encompasses not only anaesthesia but also a large element of medicine; thus where explanations for answers are not available by cross referencing the *Textbook of Anaesthesia*, we have referenced a standard textbook of medicine, *Davidson's Principles and Practice of Medicine*, 15th edition by J MacLeod, C Edwards and I Bouchier, and where extensive pharmacological and therapeutic questions are addressed we have referenced *British National Formulary* 1990 No. 20.

We must express our gratitude for the help of many colleagues and candidates from the Departments of Anaesthesia in which the authors are currently based and also in particular thank Ms Karen Marden, Principal Secretary in the University Department of Anaesthesia at Leicester for substantial secretarial work.

We hope that this text will fulfill its objectives in helping candidates to read and prepare for the FCAnaes examination and provide practice in appropriate MCQ tests.

Leicester, Warwick and Nottingham, 1990.

D.F.
D.R.D.
A.R.A.
G.S.

Introduction

There are many MCQ tutors and primers which provide practice for prospective examination candidates. Some books arrange MCQ questions under topic headings and others provide topics in random order. The latter system is similar to an actual examination with topics changing from question to question and in degree of difficulty. However, whilst this system mimics the examination, it may not be conducive to efficient learning, when candidates normally study textbooks systematically.

In this book, we have used both approaches. In the first four sections we have classified topics into physiology, pharmacology, medicine and anaesthesia, each containing 100 questions. In addition, in the final two sections, we have provided mock test papers which consist of 60 questions on a mixture of subjects in order to mimic the format of an examination paper. In all sections, we have arranged questions on the left side of the paper with answers and a brief explanation on the right in order to permit ease of checking; self-testing may be undertaken by the simple expedient of covering the right-hand page whilst reading the question stems.

In the two test papers, the overall score should provide an indication of the reader's performance; although the pass mark varies from examination to examination, the reader should hope to achieve 40% whilst 60% represents a very good mark.

The candidate should have a strategy for attempting MCQs in the examination. There are many texts which provide valuable advice and the following recommendations may be familiar. Each MCQ consists of a stem and five options or statements with a possible answer of 'true' or 'false'. In all parts of the FCAnaes examination, the MCQs are marked with a positive mark for a correct response, whilst a mark is deducted for an incorrect response and zero is given where there is no response. Thus for each stem, the range of scores varies from –5 to +5. The negative marking system should not concern you unduly. The effect is the same as scoring +2 for correct, +1 for don't know and 0 for wrong; the only difference is the position of the pass mark! Clearly, it is most unwise to guess at an answer; if you do not know the answer, you should leave it blank. Read questions carefully, and in an actual examination, take care when transferring your answers from the question paper to the computer marking sheet; it is a good idea to check each five or ten questions to ensure that your answers are not out of phase with the questions.

Practising MCQs is difficult for several reasons. Firstly, there is difficulty in finding 'examination equivalent' questions. Many trainees ask colleagues to remember questions from previous examinations and it is not unknown for departments to build up a stock of questions. However, the FCAnaes examination is reviewed continuously and the bank of questions changes constantly. Secondly, there is difficulty in defining correct answers. There are only two allowable options, 'true' or 'false' but there is no provision for 'sometimes' which enters the thought processes of both examiners and candidates not infrequently! If this occurs to the candidate, we suggest that help may be forthcoming by considering the question in a different format. For example, if a question asks if a condition is associated with certain other processes, the candidate should ask himself if these processes are clinically important or unimportant – if not, the answer is more likely to be negative.

Throughout this text, we have been brief in our explanations because providing a full explanation might have resulted in a textbook in itself! By referencing one of only three readily available books, we trust that impetus will be given to readers to consolidate their knowledge from these texts.

Abbreviations
The following abbreviations are employed in the answer sections:

A & S   Aitkenhead A R, Smith G 1990 Textbook of Anaesthesia 2nd edn. Churchill Livingstone, Edinburgh (Ch indicates the relevant chapter number; Appx indicates the relevant appendix number)

D   Macleod I, Edwards C, Bouchier I 1987 Davidson's Principles and Practice of Medicine 15th edn. Churchill Livingstone, Edinburgh (Ch indicates the relevant chapter number)

BNF   British National Formulary 20, September 1990. British Medical Association and the Pharmaceutical Society (Ch indicates the relevant chapter number; Ch Em = Emergency Treatment of Poisoning; Gui = Guidance on Prescribing)

D.F.
D.R.D.

Contents

1. Physiology

1   Functional residual capacity (FRC)

    a Represents about 75% of vital capacity.
    b May be measured by nitrogen washout.
    c Is increased in the elderly.
    d Is increased in the supine position.
    e Is always greater than closing volume.

2   Aldosterone acts to

    a Reduce Na^+ absorption in the proximal convoluted tubule.

    b Reduce Na^+ diffusion in the descending loop of Henle.

    c Increase Na^+ absorption in the distal convoluted tubule.

    d Reduce Na^+ absorption in the distal convoluted tubule.
    e Increase Na^+ absorption in the collecting ducts.

3   Albumin

    a Has a molecular weight of approximately 70 000 daltons.
    b Has a plasma concentration of 35–45 g/litre.

    c Concentration is increased in chronic liver disease.
    d Concentration is increased in malabsorption syndrome.
    e Is a major contributor to plasma oncotic pressure.

a False Normally, FRC is less than 50% of vital capacity.
b True But helium dilution is used more commonly.
c True There is loss of elastic tissue in the lungs of the elderly.
d False FRC is decreased when supine.
e False Closing volume may exceed FRC in the elderly and in the supine position.

(Ch. 4, A & S; Ch. 11, D)

a False Approximately two-thirds of the filtered sodium load is absorbed actively and passively in the proximal convoluted tubule; this is not influenced by aldosterone.
b False The descending limb of the loop of Henle is freely permeable to water, sodium and chloride and not under the influence of aldosterone.
c True This is the main action of aldosterone. Excretion of potassium ions is increased.
d False See above.
e True Sodium conservation occurs also in the collecting ducts in response to aldosterone.

(Ch. 4, A & S)

a True
b True Albumin comprises the major portion of plasma protein concentration. (Appx. III, A & S)
c False The serum albumin concentration is low in chronic liver disease.
d False Hypoalbuminaemia is likely and results in oedema.
e True Oncotic pressure in the normal individual represents the osmotic pressure of plasma proteins of which albumin is the major part.

4   The oxyhaemoglobin dissociation curve (ODC) is shifted to the left by

   a   Acidosis.

   b   The presence of carbon monoxide.

   c   Hypercapnia.
   d   Decrease in temperature.
   e   Reduced concentration of 2,3-diphosphoglyceric acid (2,3-DPG).

5   Normal atmospheric pressure is approximately

   a   760 mmHg.
   b   1000 kPa.
   c   1000 cmH$_2$O.
   d   1000 millibars.
   e   15 lb/in^2.

6   Stroke volume

   a   Is a determinant of cardiac output.
   b   Is unaffected by preload.

   c   Is related normally to afterload.

   d   Is determined normally by heart rate.

   e   Is independent of myocardial contractility.

7   Which of the following are true?

   a   The spinal cord ends at the tenth thoracic (T10) vertebral level.
   b   The subarachnoid space ends at the fifth sacral (S5) vertebral level.
   c   The dermatomal level of the costal margin in the mid clavicular line is T8.
   d   The dermatomal level of the lateral aspect of the elbow is C5.
   e   The dermatomal level of the nipples is T2.

(Ch. 2, A & S)

a False The ODC is shifted to the right by increased temperature, hydrogen ion concentration, carbon dioxide tension and 2, 3-diphosphoglyceric acid concentration. Decreases in these variables cause a leftward shift of the ODC.
b True Carbon monoxide combines with haemoglobin to form carboxyhaemoglobin, reducing the total capacity of blood to carry oxygen.
c False See **a**.
d True See **a**.
e True See **a**. 2, 3-DPG concentration is reduced in stored blood.

(Ch. 16, A & S)

a True
b False It is 101.3 kPa.
c True
d True
e True

(Ch. 3, A & S)

a True Cardiac output = heart rate × stroke volume.
b False Stroke volume is proportional to preload. This is the Frank-Starling law.
c False However, in the failing ventricle stroke volume decreases with increasing afterload.
d False But at very high heart rates there is decreased ventricular filling time and stroke volume may decrease.
e False There is a direct relationship.

(Ch. 1, A & S)

a False The spinal cord ends normally at L1.
b False The subarachnoid space extends in the adult to S2.

c True

d True *(Ch. 26, A & S)*
e False The level is T4.

8   Systemic arterial pressure is increased
- **a** On assumption of the erect from the supine position.
- **b** On sudden exposure to cold.
- **c** Always when heart rate increases.
- **d** By carotid sinus hypoxia.
- **e** In response to stimulation by peripheral chemoreceptors.

9   Carbon dioxide is transported in the blood mostly
- **a** As carboxyhaemoglobin.
- **b** In combination with plasma protein.
- **c** As bicarbonate.
- **d** Dissolved in plasma as carbonic acid.
- **e** At a partial pressure of 5.3 kPa in mixed venous blood.

10   Which statements are true of cranial nerves?
- **a** The vagus supplies all the intrinsic muscles of the larynx.
- **b** All intrinsic muscles of the tongue are supplied by the hypoglossal nerve.
- **c** All extrinsic muscles of the tongue are supplied by cranial nerves.
- **d** The baroreceptors are innervated by the cranial root of the accessory nerve.
- **e** The glossopharyngeal subserves sensation from the posterior third of the tongue and all of the epiglottis.

11   During pregnancy
- **a** Plasma osmolality is increased.
- **b** Plasma cholinesterase concentration is increased.
- **c** There is an increase in functional residual capacity (FRC).
- **d** Haemoglobin concentration is decreased.
- **e** Absorption of calcium ions via the gut is increased.

(Ch. 3, A & S)

a False Arterial pressure tends to decrease initially.
b True Because of peripheral vasoconstriction.
c False This increases cardiac output but does not necessarily influence systemic arterial pressure.
d False Systemic arterial pressure is increased in response to relaxation of tension in the walls of the carotid sinus, not hypoxaemia.
e True Stimulation of peripheral chemoreceptors mainly causes hyperventilation.

(Ch. 2, A & S)

a False Carboxyhaemoglobin is the compound formed by combination of carbon monoxide with haemoglobin.
b False Combination of carbon dioxide with plasma proteins does not occur.
c True This involves ionisation of carbonic acid and the chloride shift.
d False Carbonic acid dissociates into hydrogen ions and bicarbonate ions.
e False The partial pressure of carbon dioxide is about 6 kPa in mixed venous blood.

(Ch. 1, A & S)

a True Via the superior and recurrent laryngeal nerves.
b True

c True
d False Impulses from baroreceptors are carried in the carotid sinus nerve, a branch of the glossopharyngeal nerve.
e False The posterior part of the epiglottis is innervated by the vagus nerve.

(Ch. 6, A & S)

a False Osmolality decreases although aldosterone secretion increases because of a resistance which develops to the action of mineralocorticoids.
b False Plasma cholinesterase concentration is decreased.
c False FRC is decreased in pregnancy as a result of a decrease in residual volume.
d True Plasma volume increases more than the increase in red cell mass, with a resultant decrease in haemoglobin concentration.
e False Absorption capacity for calcium is unchanged. The increased needs of pregnancy may result in calcium deficiency.

12   The sacral canal
a   Contains the filum terminale.
b   Contains the epidural plexus of veins.
c   Is lined with dura mater.

d   Has five intervertebral foramina.

e   The meninges end at S2.

13   In comparison with intracellular fluid, extracellular fluid has
a   Greater volume.

b   Greater potassium concentration.

c   Lower bicarbonate concentration.
d   Greater chloride concentration.
e   Greater osmolality.

14   Glucagon
a   Is secreted by the beta cells of the pancreas.

b   Increases free fatty acid concentration in blood.

c   Is secreted in response to hyperglycaemia.
d   Stimulates the secretion of insulin.

e   Increases glycogenolysis.

15   Catecholamine release is stimulated by the following
a   Hypoxaemia.

b   Hypothermia.

c   Hypoglycaemia.

d   Hypercapnia.

e   Hypocalcaemia.

(Ch. 1, A & S)

a True
b True The extradural space extends to the sacral hiatus.
c False The sacral canal is not usually lined with dura mater. In the adult, this normally terminates at approximately the second sacral segment, where it becomes the filum terminale.
d False The five sacral nerves exit through bilateral intervertebral foramina. Thus, there are 10!
e True But they may extend further in the neonate.

(Ch. 4, A & S)

a False Total body water comprises approximately 60% of body weight; two-thirds of the water is intracellular.
b False Potassium forms the major intracellular cation with a concentration of approximately 150 mmol/litre.
c False
d True Chloride is present in cells in a concentration of only 10 mmol/litre.
e False Osmolality is similar in extracellular and intracellular fluids.

(Ch. 9, Ch. 12, D)

a False Glucagon is secreted by the alpha cells of the pancreas. Beta cells produce insulin.
b True The actions of glucagon oppose those of insulin; lipolysis is stimulated, releasing free fatty acids.
c False Hyperglycaemia inhibits glucagon release.
d True Glucagon stimulates the release of insulin by a local effect in the pancreas.
e True Glycogenolysis results in an increase in blood glucose concentration.

a True The tachycardia associated with hypoxaemia is secondary to sympatho adrenal activity.
b False Hypothermia reduces basal metabolic rate and catecholamine secretion. *(Ch. 23, A & S)*
c True Hypoglycaemia stimulates catecholamine release, producing the characteristic signs of sweating and tachycardia. *(Ch. 12, D)*
d True Carbon dioxide retention stimulates catecholamine release. *(Ch. 42, A & S)*
e False There is no effect of hypocalcaemia on the sympathoadrenal axis. *(Ch. 5, A & S)*

16   Insulin causes

a   Reduced gluconeogenesis.

b   Increased glycogenolysis.

c   Synthesis of proteins from amino acids.

d   Entry of potassium into cells.
e   Lipolysis.

17   Severing the cervical sympathetic trunk results in

a   Dilatation of the pupil.
b   Reduction in sweating.
c   Partial ptosis.

d   Decreased taste sensation on the anterior two-thirds of the tongue.
e   Dry oral mucous membrane.

18   The following occur postoperatively

a   Increased secretion of ADH.

b   Increased loss of potassium.

c   Decreased loss of sodium.
d   Decreased urine osmolality.

e   Increased FRC.

19   Alveolar P_{CO_2} (PA_{CO_2})

a   Has a normal range of 4.8–5.8 kPa.
b   Differs from arterial P_{CO_2} by 1–1.5 kPa.
c   Is reduced by increased minute ventilation.
d   Is identical in value to mixed venous P_{CO_2}.
e   Is similar in value to end-tidal CO_2.

(Ch. 12, D)

a True Insulin causes glucose uptake by the cell and inhibits gluconeogenesis.
b False Glycogenolysis is the breakdown of glycogen to starch and sugar. This is inhibited by insulin.
c True Insulin is an anabolic hormone. The absence of insulin leads to protein breakdown.
d True Reduced plasma concentrations of insulin lead to hyperkalaemia.
e False Lack of insulin leads to lipolysis.

(Ch. 15, D)

a False Pupillary constriction – miosis occurs.
b True Anhidrosis is part of Horner's syndrome.
c True The levator palpebrae superioris is innervated partly by the sympathetic system in addition to the seventh cranial nerve.
d False Taste on the anterior two-thirds of the tongue is subserved by the lingual nerve – a branch of the mandibular nerve.
e False The secretomotor supply to the mucous membrane is parasympathetic in origin.

---

a True Increased production of ADH occurs postoperatively as part of the normal endocrine response to stress.
b True Increased serum cortisol concentration caused by stress leads to retention of sodium and water and loss of potassium ions. *(Ch. 12, D)*
c True See **b**.
d False Because of sodium and water retention and the effect of ADH, urine osmolality postoperatively is greater than normal.
e False FRC is reduced intraoperatively because of increased activity of muscles of expiration and cranial displacement of the diaphragm. In addition, FRC may be reduced after abdominal or thoracic surgery because of pain and splinting of the diaphragm. *(Ch. 2, A & S)*

(Ch. 2, A & S)

a True This reflects arterial P_{CO_2}. *(Appx. XI, A & S)*
b False
c True The relationship is hyperbolic.
d False Alveolar P_{CO_2} is equal to arterial P_{CO_2} in the normal patient.
e True End-tidal CO_2 approximates to alveolar P_{CO_2} in healthy lungs, but is lower in patients with increased V/Q mismatch.

20   Intestinal motor activity
  a   Is inhibited by gastrin.
  b   Is increased by vagal stimulation.
  c   Is increased by sympathetic block.

  d   Is increased by moderate distension.

  e   Is diminished during labour.

21   In the kidney
  a   Most sodium is absorbed in the proximal tubule.
  b   Glucose is not excreted if the serum glucose concentration is normal.
  c   Tubular cells secrete ammonium ions.

  d   Acetazolamide acts on tubular production of HCO_3^-.

  e   Aldosterone is secreted by the juxtaglomerular apparatus.

22   At the start of a forced expiration against a closed glottis there is
  a   Increased intrathoracic pressure.

  b   Increased systolic arterial pressure.

  c   Increased heart rate.

  d   Raised right ventricular output

  e   Decrease in left ventricular output.

23   Gastric emptying is accelerated by
  a   Erect posture.
  b   Gastrin.

  c   Cholecystokinin.

  d   Increased osmotic pressure of the duodenal contents.
  e   Secretin.

a **False**
b **True**
c **True** Sympathetic block permits unopposed action of the parasympathetic nervous system. *(Ch. 26, A & S)*
d **True** Distension of the gut causes reflex stimulation of intestinal activity. However, activity is decreased in the presence of gross distension.
e **True** Gastrointestinal activity is diminished during pregnancy and labour. *(Ch. 6, A & S)*

(Ch. 4, A & S)

a **True** 70% of sodium absorption occurs in the proximal tubule.
b **True** Provided that the renal threshold for glucose is normal, glycosuria does not occur unless hyperglycaemia is present.
c **True** Tubular secretion of ammonium ions facilitates hydrogen ion excretion and bicarbonate conservation.
d **True** Acetazolamide is a carbonic anhydrase inhibitor which interferes with bicarbonate reabsorption.
e **False** The juxtaglomerular apparatus is responsible for renin production; the renin-angiotensin system is responsible for aldosterone secretion.

(Ch. 3, A & S)

a **True** The Valsalva manoeuvre produces an increased intrathoracic pressure.
b **True** There is a transient increase in systolic arterial pressure due to increased ejection from the left ventricle.
c **False** There is an initial transient decrease in heart rate with the Valsalva manoeuvre.
d **True** There is an initial increase in right ventricular output followed rapidly by a decrease as venous return into the thorax is impeded.
e **False** There is an initial increase in left ventricular output followed rapidly by a decrease in overall cardiac output.

(Ch. 32, A & S; Ch. 9, D)

a **True** Assumption of the erect posture enhances gastric emptying.
b **False** Gastrin is secreted by the gastric antrum and stimulates the secretion of gastric acid and pepsin.
c **False** Cholecystokinin is secreted in response to duodenal stimulation and inhibits gastric emptying.
d **False** This is part of the enterogastric reflex.
e **False** Secretin is released in parallel with cholecystokinin.

24   In the conducting system of the heart

   a   The sino-atrial node is situated in the wall of the right atrium.

   b   The normal resting potential of cardiac muscle is -80 to -90 mV.

   c   The PR interval represents the duration of atrial depolarisation.
   d   The normal PR interval is greater than 0.2 s.
   e   Atrial conduction is slowed by a decrease in temperature.

25   The following are true

   a   Sodium is the main determinant of extracellular fluid osmolality.

   b   Hypernatraemia results in intracellular dehydration.

   c K^+ is the main determinant of intracellular osmolality.

   d   Acidosis increases intracellular K^+.

   e   The combination of a low ECF chloride and normal sodium concentration indicates respiratory alkalosis.

26   Lung compliance

   a   Is the reciprocal of airways resistance.

   b   Is expressed as cmH_2O/litre.
   c   Is increased in the presence of emphysema.
   d   Is increased in the presence of pulmonary oedema.

   e   Is unaffected by anaesthesia.

27   CSF normally has a

   a   Protein content of 200 mg/litre

   b P_{CO_2} higher than that of arterial blood.

   c   Specific gravity of 1040.
   d   A pressure of 100 mm of CSF.

   e   Volume of about 60 ml in an average adult.

(Ch. 3, A & S)

a True The sino-atrial node lies in the wall of the right atrium close to the superior vena cava.

b True The resting membrane potential is determined by the relative concentrations of potassium as described by the Nernst equation. *(Ch. 5, A & S)*

c False Atrial depolarisation is represented by the P wave.

d False The normal PR interval is 0.12–0.20 s. *(Appx. IV, A & S)*

e True A decrease in temperature decreases cellular activity including depolarisation.

(Ch. 22, Appx. VI, A & S)

a True ECF osmolality is normally approximately 300 mosm/kg; sodium accounts for approx. 145 mosm/kg.

b True Water moves along an osmotic gradient from intracellular to extracellular compartments.

c True Intracellular potassium concentration is approximately 150 mmol/litre.

d False In acidosis, there is a shift in potassium from the intracellular to the extracellular compartment.

e False Chronic respiratory acidosis may result in hypochloraemia secondary to compensatory bicarbonate conservation.

(Ch. 2, A & S)

a False Units of compliance contain no time base in contrast to those of resistance.

b False It is expressed as change in volume/change in pressure (litre/kPa).

c False Emphysema results in loss of elastic tissue in the lungs.

d False The lungs are less compliant (stiffer) if pulmonary oedema is present.

e False Compliance decreases during anaesthesia.

(Ch. 5, A & S)

a True Protein content is lower than that in plasma but may be increased in conditions such as Guillain-Barré syndrome.

b False Carbon dioxide diffuses readily between CSF and blood but is buffered less efficiently in CSF; thus, acute changes produce large changes in CSF pH.

c False Specific gravity is approximately 1005.

d True With the patient lying in the lateral position, the pressure range is normally 5–15 cm of CSF. *(Ch. 15, D)*

e False Volume is approximately 120 ml and the CSF undergoes rapid (4-hourly) turnover.

28 **The following are true of fluid balance**

    a The fluid requirement of a 15 kg child is 3.5 ml/kg per hour.

    b Insensible daily loss for a 70 kg man in a normal environment is more than 1200 ml.

    c Obligatory daily urine production in a normal environment for a 70 kg man is more than 800 ml.

    d The total body water of infants and small children is approximately 80% of body weight.

    e Total body water of infants and small children is 80 ml/kg body weight.

---

29 **With respect to the circulation in a healthy adult**

    a The major proportion of blood volume is accommodated in the low–pressure venous circulation.

    b A decrease of up to 15% of blood volume is compensated for by an increase in vasomotor tone.

    c A 10% decrease in blood volume results in a reduction in cardiac output.

    d Arterial pressure is not a good index of blood loss.

    e CVP decreases in response to a 10% reduction in circulating blood volume.

---

30 **With respect to renal physiology**

    a About 200 litres of water are filtered daily through the glomeruli.

    b Sodium filtration through the glomeruli is about 30 000 mmol/24 h.

    c Glomerular filtration rate (GFR) is constant over a wide range of systemic arterial pressures.

    d Normally, 90% of glomerular filtrate is reabsorbed.

    e Normally, at least 98% of filtered sodium is reabsorbed by the proximal tubules.

(Ch. 32, A & S)

a True This child requires (4 × 10 ml/h) + (2 × 5 ml/h) = 50 ml/h.
(Appx. IX, A & S)
b False In a temperate climate, up to one litre of water daily may be lost in
expired air and by evaporation. (Ch. 5, D)
c False Urine osmolality may reach a maximum of 1200–1400 mosmol/kg;
with a normal diet, the minimum volume of urine required is about
500 ml. (Ch. 4, A & S; Ch. 11, D)
d True This varies from 75–85% of body weight and exceeds the value for
an adult.
e False This is the blood volume of infants and small children.

(Ch. 32, A & S)

a True The veins contain approximately 80% of the blood volume.
(Ch. 3, A & S)
b True However, when more than 15% of the intravascular volume is lost,
tachycardia and orthostatic hypotension develop.
c False Most healthy adults can cope with a 10% decrease in intravascular
volume with no change in cardiac output.
d True However, in the elderly and those with compromised circulatory
reflexes, there is less tolerance to small decreases in blood volume.
e False However, with loss of intravascular volume in excess of 10%, a
decrease in CVP occurs.

(Ch. 4, A & S; Ch. 11, D)

a True Water and substances of small molecular weight pass through the
glomerular capillary wall.
b True Sodium passes through the glomerular capillary wall. The normal
plasma sodium concentration (150 mmol/litre) multiplied by the 24 h
filtration rate (200 litre/24 h) gives a value of about 30 000 mmol.
c True Cortical autoregulation maintains GFR constant over a range of
arterial pressures from 90–180 mmHg.
d False Normally, 99% of glomerular filtrate is reabsorbed by the renal
tubules.
e False Although at least 98% of filtered sodium is absorbed in the kidney,
the proximal tubule accounts for approximately 70%.

31   A serum sodium concentration of 142 mmol/litre, and serum potassium concentration of 6.2 mmol/litre are compatible with

a   Hypopituitarism.

b   Addison's disease.
c   Persistent severe hypovolaemia.

d   Myxoedema.
e   Stored CPD blood.

32   Aldosterone

a   Is a polypeptide.

b   Is synthesised in the zona glomerulosa of the adrenal cortex.
c   Acts on the proximal tubule of the kidney.

d   Increases urinary [K$^+$].

e   Decreases urinary pH.

33   Antidiuretic hormone (ADH)

a   Decreases the permeability of the collecting ducts of the kidney.

b   Acts via cyclic AMP.

c   Is secreted in response to neural stimuli originating in the hypothalamus.
d   Is secreted in response to hypovolaemia even if plasma is hypotonic.
e   Is secreted in response to pain and stress.

(Ch. 12, D)

a False Secretion of aldosterone is unaltered in hypopituitarism, and therefore potassium excretion is not usually abnormal.

b False Hyponatraemia is normally a feature of Addison's disease.

c True In severe circulatory failure there is impairment of potassium excretion by the kidney, and potassium may be released from cells damaged by trauma.

d False

e True Hyperkalaemia occurs in stored blood. The serum potassium concentration may increase to this value within a few days of storage. *(Ch. 7, A & S)*

(Ch. 4, A & S)

a False Aldosterone is a mineralocorticoid with a steroid structure. *(Ch. 12, D)*

b True The zona glomerulosa is the outermost layer of the adrenal cortex.

c False Aldosterone acts on the distal tubule to cause retention of sodium and excretion of potassium.

d True Potassium and/or hydrogen ions are secreted into the tubule in exchange for reabsorbed sodium. Thus, urinary potassium and hydrogen ion secretion are enhanced.

e False Although aldosterone increases tubular secretion of hydrogen ions, these are buffered.

(Ch. 4, A & S)

a False ADH increases the permeability of the collecting ducts to water. Thus urine volume is decreased.

b True Cyclic AMP acts as a second messenger.

c True Osmoreceptors in the hypothalamus detect changes in plasma osmolality.

d True ADH is part of the endocrine response to stress and this overrides osmolar regulation.

e True See above.

34   The sodium-potassium pump at the cell membrane

  a   Requires ATP.

  b   Is inhibited by ouabain.

  c   Maintains a low intracellular chloride concentration.

  d   Is responsible for active transport of sodium ions into the cell.

  e   Is responsible for generation of action potentials.

35   Renal blood flow

  a   Is subject to autoregulation.

  b   Is greater in the renal cortex than in the medulla.

  c   May be measured using the Fick principle.

  d   Is approximately 10% of cardiac output.

  e   Is unaltered by haemorrhagic shock.

36   Active transport is involved in transfer across renal cell membranes of

  a   Potassium ions.

  b   Sodium ions.

  c   Glucose.

  d   Amino acids.

  e   Protein.

(Ch. 5, A & S)

a True Ion movement across the cell membrane occurs against an electrochemical gradient and therefore requires energy.

b True In common with other cardiac glycosides, ouabain increases the concentration of intracellular calcium by inhibition of sodium-potassium exchange at the cell membrane. *(Ch. 14, A & S)*

c False The cell membrane is permeable to chloride which diffuses along an electrochemical gradient from intracellular to extracellular fluid.

d False Sodium is transported from inside to outside the cell against its concentration gradient.

e False The sodium-potassium pump is responsible for maintenance of the resting membrane potential and for repolarising the membrane after depolarisation by an action potential.

(Ch. 4, A & S)

a True Autoregulation maintains constant renal blood flow in the face of changing perfusion pressure (within limits).

b True Autoregulation occurs in the cortex but not in the medulla. The afferent arteriole dilates when arterial pressure is decreased.

c True The Fick principle states that uptake or clearance of a substance by an organ is equal to its arterio-venous content difference multiplied by blood flow through the organ. In this case, para-aminohippuric acid (PAH) is used as the tracer substance.

d False The blood flow to the kidney is approximately 25% of cardiac output.

e False In haemorrhagic shock, medullary perfusion is impaired and, if blood pressure decreases below the lower limit of autoregulation, cortical perfusion is reduced also.

(Ch. 11, D)

a True Active sodium/potassium exchange occurs in the distal tubule and collecting duct.

b True In addition to **a** above, sodium is reabsorbed actively in the proximal tubule.

c True Almost 100% of glucose is reabsorbed by the proximal tubule unless T_{max} is exceeded. *(Ch. 4, A & S)*

d True Amino acids are transported actively out of the tubular lumen in the proximal tubule.

e False Protein does not appear in the glomerular filtrate under normal circumstances.

37 **Which of the following are consistent with acute renal tubular necrosis?**

   a Oliguria.

   b A normal cortical blood flow.

   c Increased urine urea concentration.

   d Hyperkalaemia.

   e Oedema.

38 **A serum osmolality of 360 mosmol/kg is compatible with**

   a Excessive secretion of ADH.

   b Normal serum.

   c Uraemia.

   d Fresh-water drowning.

   e Uncontrolled diabetes mellitus.

39 **Inulin**

   a Is cleared completely from blood in a single passage through the kidney.

   b Is not reabsorbed from glomerular filtrate.

   c Is present in glomerular filtrate in a concentration equal to that in plasma.

   d Is secreted by the renal tubules.

   e Does not pass into the extravascular space.

40 **Soluble insulin**

   a Increases the entry of glucose into muscle cells.

   b Induces protein catabolism.

   c Increases the transport of amino acids into cells.

   d Is a polypeptide secreted by the alpha cells of the islets of Langerhans.

   e Has a duration of action of 12 h when given by subcutaneous injection.

(Ch. 11, D)

a True Oliguria is a feature of acute tubular necrosis.
b False There is reduction in blood flow to the cortex.
c False Urinary urea concentration is decreased because of reduced GFR and impaired tubular function.
d True There is impaired ability to excrete potassium, and hyperkalaemia may require treatment with intravenous insulin and glucose.
e True Pulmonary oedema is a serious complication and may be caused by excessive administration of intravenous fluids.

---

a False Excessive secretion of ADH results in water retention and a decrease in serum osmolality. *(Ch. 5, D.)*
b False Normal serum osmolality is 280–300 mosmol/kg. *(Appx. III, A & S)*
c True Urea contributes to serum osmolality.
d False Absorption of inhaled water is likely to lead to reduction in concentration of plasma constituents.
e True Hyperosmolar non-ketotic coma may occur especially in the elderly diabetic. *(Ch. 12, D)*

(Ch. 4, A & S)

a True Inulin clearance represents glomerular filtration rate.

b True Because it is not reabsorbed from glomerular filtrate, its clearance represents GFR.

c True Because inulin is cleared in a single passage through the glomerulus, the concentration in the glomerular filtrate is equal to that in plasma. It should be noted that inulin has to be infused i.v. to achieve a steady plasma concentration.
d False It is neither absorbed nor secreted by the kidney tubules.
e False Inulin is a polymer with molecular weight 5000, and passes readily through capillary membranes into the extravascular space.

(Ch. 12, D)

a True This is the prime action of this endocrine hormone.
b False Insulin is an anabolic hormone which stimulates fat and protein synthesis. During the catabolic (stress) response to trauma and surgery, secretion of insulin is suppressed.
c False Insulin facilitates the entry of glucose but not amino acids into cells.
d False Insulin is a polypeptide which is secreted by the beta cells of the islets of Langerhans.
e False The duration of action of soluble insulin is approximately 6 h.
(Ch. 41, A & S)

41   Cardiac muscle differs from skeletal muscle in that it
a   Has a longer refractory period.
b   Depolarises spontaneously.
c   Can metabolise lactic acid.
d   Can only contract isometrically.
e   Has a low extraction ratio for oxygen.

42   Haemoglobin
a   Is a mucopolysaccharide.
b   Binds four molecules of oxygen per molecule.
c   Has a theoretical oxygen carrying capacity of 1.34 mlO_2/g.
d   Is catabolised in the reticulo-endothelial system (RES).
e   Is an important buffer in the blood.

43   Plasma volume may be measured using
a   Para-aminohippuric acid.
b   Inulin.
c   Radio-labelled albumin.
d   Evans blue.
e   Creatinine.

44   The P_{50}
a   Is increased by violent exercise.
b   Is increased when blood pH decreases.
c   Is unaffected by the operation of the Bohr effect.
d   Is increased by increase in 2, 3-DPG concentration in the erythrocytes.
e   Is increased during ascent to high altitudes.

(Ch. 3, A & S)

a True Because of calcium influx, the period of depolarisation (and therefore the refractory period) is prolonged.

b True The phase zero pre-potential of cardiac muscle reflects leakage of sodium ions into the cell and a decrease in the leakage of potassium ions out of the cell. At a potential of -50 mV, spontaneous depolarisation occurs.

c False Lactic acid may be produced in a hypoxic environment but is not metabolised.

d False There is an isotonic phase of contraction as well as an isometric phase.

e False The extraction ratio of cardiac muscle is very high. The blood returning into the coronary sinus is amongst the most desaturated found in the body. Coronary venous P_{O_2} is approximately 4 kPa.

(Ch. 13, D; Ch. 2, A & S)

a False Haemoglobin is a protein.

b True The affinity of each haem fraction for each molecule of oxygen varies with the occupation of the other oxygen-carrying sites. It is this characteristic of haemoglobin to facilitate oxygen uptake which results in the sigmoid oxyhaemoglobin dissociation curve.

c False The theoretical oxygen-carrying capacity of haemoglobin (Hufner's constant) is 1.39 ml/g, but the experimental value is 1.34 ml/g.

d True The principal catabolic site of haemoglobin is the monocyte-macrophage system (formerly RES) of the liver and spleen.

e True Haemoglobin is a very important buffer system in peripheral blood. *(Ch. 2, A & S)*

(Ch. 4, A & S)

a False Para-aminohippuric acid is one of the substances used to measure renal plasma flow.

b False Inulin is used to measure glomerular filtration rate.

c True Iodine-labelled albumin may be used.

d True Evans blue may be used for a dye dilution technique. *(Ch. 3, A & S)*

e False Creatinine is used to measure glomerular filtration rate.

(Ch. 2, A & S)

a True Violent exercise causes an increase in body temperature and this shifts the oxyhaemoglobin dissociation curve (ODC) to the right, causing an increase in the P_{50}.

b True This shifts the ODC to the right.

c False The Bohr effect is a shift to the right with increasing hydrogen ion concentration.

d True 2, 3-DPG is produced by glycolysis; this shifts the ODC to the right, thus increasing the P_{50}.

e False Ascent to altitude induces acute hyperventilation with decrease in P_{CO_2} and a consequent shift of the ODC to the left. *(Ch. 18, D)*

45 The Frank-Starling mechanism

a Relates force of contraction to fibre length.

b Does not operate in the human heart.

c Operates only in the denervated heart.

d Is abolished by changes in contractility.

e Is unaffected by afterload.

46 Cardiac output

a May increase to values of 35 litre/min during exercise.
b Is increased by vagal stimulation.

c Is uninfluenced by infusion of noradrenaline.

d Is increased by administration of adrenaline.
e Is increased when contractility increases.

47 Pulmonary blood flow

a Is distributed equally throughout the lungs.

b Is decreased by sympathetic stimulation.

c Is unchanged during exercise.

d Is not influenced by changes in alveolar P_{O_2}.

e Is abnormal in the presence of significant pulmonary embolus.

48 In an ECG trace

a The paper speed is normally 2.5 cm/s.
b The PR interval is measured from the peak of the P wave to the peak of the R wave.
c The T wave becomes more peaked as the serum K^+ concentration increases.
d Left ventricular hypertrophy is present when R in V_5 or V_6 plus S in V_1 is greater than 40 mm (4 mV).
e P waves are absent in atrial flutter.

(Ch. 3, A & S)

a True The Frank-Starling mechanism states that force of contraction is determined by the initial fibre length.

b False Although originally described in animals, the principle may be applied in man. Indirect indices of fibre length (e.g., LVEDP) are used.

c False The mechanism operates in the denervated heart and also under normal circumstances.

d False Changes in contractility merely move the position of the curve relating contractility to initial fibre length.

e False Afterload affects LVEDP, and therefore initial fibre length.

(Ch. 3, A & S)

a True This occurs predominantly because of an increase in stroke volume.

b False Increased vagal tone decreases heart rate and, to a certain extent, contractility.

c False Noradrenaline increases afterload causing decreases in heart rate and cardiac output. However, it may also exert an agonist action at beta-receptors and in some circumstances increase cardiac output.

d True Adrenaline has positive inotropic and chronotropic actions.

e True Cardiac output depends upon heart rate and stroke volume. Stroke volume is increased with increasing contractility.

(Ch. 2, A & S)

a False 60% of right ventricular output is distributed to the lower 40% of lung volume in the erect position because of the influence of gravity.

b False Sympathetic stimulation increases cardiac output and pulmonary blood flow.

c False Exercise-induced increases in cardiac output result in an increase in pulmonary blood flow.

d False A decrease in alveolar P_{O_2} causes hypoxic pulmonary vasoconstriction (HPV). This reflex is attenuated by inhalational anaesthetics. *(Ch. 39, A & S)*

e True The greater the size of an embolus, the greater proportion of the pulmonary circulation is occluded.

(Ch. 7, D)

a True This is the conventional speed for ECG recording.

b False The PR interval is measured from the beginning of the P wave to the beginning of the R wave.

c True Tall, tented T waves are characteristic of hyperkalaemia.

d True

e True P waves represent atrial depolarisation in sinus rhythm. Flutter waves are present in the condition of atrial flutter.

49 **The following are true for a blood sample with a P_{O_2} of 6.0 kPa**

    a It is arterial blood; mean V/Q ratio is less than normal.

    b It is venous blood from a normal patient.
    c Oxygen saturation is 80% (assuming normal pH, temperature, base excess, adult blood).
    d It is 90% saturated fetal blood.

    e It may be arterial blood from a patient with 50% right-to-left shunt.

50 **Functional residual capacity**

    a Is the sum of the residual volume and the inspiratory reserve volume.

    b Is uninfluenced by posture.
    c Becomes less than closing volume with advancing age.

    d Is a measure of the resting expiratory position.

    e May be measured by the helium dilution method.

51 **The following variables are employed in the Bohr-Enghoff equation**

    a Inspired P_{CO_2}.

    b Mean expired CO_2 concentration.
    c Pc'CO_2.
    d Tidal volume.
    e Cardiac output.

52 **Upper airway obstruction**

    a Decreases maximum breathing capacity.
    b Increases functional residual capacity.

    c Decreases FEV_1.

    d Increases lung compliance.
    e May diminish air trapping.

a True This represents severe hypoxaemia which could be accounted for by a V/Q ratio less than unity.

b True Normal mixed venous P_{O_2} is 5.4 kPa. *(Ch. 3, A & S)*

c True Assuming a normal P_{50}, this would represent an oxygen saturation of 80%.

d True The oxyhaemoglobin dissociation curve of fetal haemoglobin has a lower P_{50} than that of adult haemoglobin, and a P_{O_2} of 6 kPa represents saturation of about 90%. *(Ch. 34, A & S)*

e True A 50% shunt would result in a saturation of 80–85% which corresponds to a P_{O_2} of 6 kPa, assuming a normal ODC.

a False FRC is the sum of the residual volume and expiratory reserve volume; it represents the volume in the lungs at the end of a normal tidal breath. (Appx. XI, A & S)

b False FRC is reduced in the supine position.

c True Closing volume increases with increasing age and exceeds FRC in the elderly.

d True FRC represents a balance between elastic recoil of the lungs and that of the chest wall at the end of expiration.

e True This is the standard method for measurement of FRC.

a True Inspired CO_2 constitutes part of the Bohr equation, although it is usually negligible and is commonly ignored.

b True

c False

d True

e False

a True

b False FRC is the end-expiratory position and is unrelated to upper airway obstruction – although it might be difficult to measure in the presence of obstruction.

c True FEV_1 may be measured with the Vitalograph. Upper airway obstruction decreases the ability to exhale rapidly.

d False Compliance is independent of time.

e True Partial upper airway obstruction has the same effect as positive airway pressure (CPAP)

53 **In a spontaneously breathing patient with upper respiratory obstruction, helium is beneficial because**
   a   It is the best means of improving oxygenation.
   b CO_2 elimination is achieved more easily.

   c   Its viscosity overcomes small airways obstruction.
   d   Its density overcomes large airways obstruction.

   e   It overcomes resistance in areas of laminar flow.

54 **An area in the lung with increased ventilation/perfusion ratio**
   a   Represents shunt.
   b   Represents dead space.
   c   Is responsible for a decrease in Pa_{O_2} with no change in Pa_{CO_2}.

   d   May be compensated for by increasing F_{IO_2}.

   e   May be compensated for by increased minute ventilation.

55 **Carbon dioxide retention may cause**
   a   Increase in plasma catecholamine concentrations.
   b   Sweating.
   c   Cardiac arrhythmias.

   d   Constricted pupils.

   e   Decreased cardiac output.

56 **The basilic vein**
   a   Accompanies the radial artery.
   b   Arises on the palmar aspect of the hand.
   c   Courses between the pectoralis major and the deltoid.

   d   Joins the axillary vein.
   e   Runs on the radial side of the forearm.

(Ch. 16, A & S)

a False The best way to improve oxygenation is to increase F_{IO_2}.
b True A helium/oxygen mixture improves alveolar ventilation and may delay the onset of hypercapnic respiratory failure.
c False The viscosity of helium is similar to that of oxygen.
d True The lower density of helium compared with air or oxygen results in lower resistance in an obstructed upper airway, where flow is turbulent.
e False Laminar flow depends upon gas viscosity, not density.

(Ch. 2, A & S)

a False Increased V/Q ratio constitutes increased dead space.
b True Shunting would be represented by a decreased V/Q ratio.
c False If minute ventilation remains unchanged, Pa_{CO_2} increases and Pa_{O_2} decreases. If alveolar ventilation is maintained by an increase in total minute ventilation, Pa_{CO_2} remains constant but Pa_{O_2} does not decrease.
d False Compensation occurs only by an increase in minute ventilation, although the decreased Pa_{O_2} can be overcome by increasing F_{IO_2}.
e True Increased minute ventilation is necessary to maintain alveolar ventilation in the presence of increased physiological dead space.

(Ch. 24, A & S)

a True Carbon dioxide causes an increase in sympatho-adrenal output.
b True Excessive sympatho-adrenal activity causes sweating.
c True This results from release of adrenaline and respiratory acidosis, which accompany carbon dioxide retention.
d False Dilated pupils would be expected in the presence of catecholamine secretion.
e False Carbon dioxide retention causes an increased cardiac output.

(Ch. 1, A & S)

a False The basilic vein lies on the ulnar side of the arm.
b False The basilic vein arises on the ulnar side of the wrist.
c False The cephalic vein pierces the clavipectoral fascia between pectoralis major and deltoid.
d True The basilic vein joins the axillary vein to form the subclavian vein.
e False See **a**.

57   The anterior pituitary secretes

a   Oxytocin.

b   Aldosterone.

c   Thyrotrophin.

d   Prolactin.

e   Somatostatin.

58   The sympathetic nervous system

a   Does not possess cholinergic fibres.

b   Releases hormones which may be blocked by guanethidine.

c   Inhibits motility in the gastrointestinal system.

d   Produces miosis.

e   Possesses fibres which run in the vagus nerve.

59   The knee jerk reflex

a   Is mediated via T12.

b   Is mediated via afferent impulses from receptors in the patellar tendon.

c   Is mediated via afferent impulses from receptors in the quadriceps muscle.

d   Is a monosynaptic reflex.

e   Disappears under deep general anaesthesia.

(Ch. 12, D)

a False Oxytocin is secreted by the posterior pituitary gland (neurohypophysis).
b False Aldosterone is an adrenocortical hormone secreted under the influence of the renin-angiotensin system.
c True Thyrotrophin (TSH) is secreted by the anterior pituitary under the influence of thyrotrophin releasing hormone (TRH).
d True Prolactin (PRL) is secreted under the inhibitory control of dopamine from the hypothalamus.
e False Somatostatin (GHRIH) is the inhibitory hormone from the hypothalamus which controls growth hormone secretion from the anterior pituitary.

(Ch. 5, A & S)

a False Preganglionic sympathetic fibres are cholinergic, as are sympathetic fibres to the sweat glands and some vessels in muscle.
b True Guanethidine inhibits release of noradrenaline from postganglionic fibres and also depletes the nerve endings of noradrenaline. It is used in an IVRA technique to produce peripheral sympathetic block.
c True Sympathetic stimulation decreases gastrointestinal motility and causes sphincter contraction. *(Ch. 13, A & S)*
d False Sympathetic activity results in pupillary dilation.
e True Sympathetic fibres to the heart, bronchi and gut accompany the parasympathetic vagal supply to these organs.

(Ch. 15, D)

a False The knee jerk reflex is mediated via L3–4.
b False Stretching the patellar tendon activates stretch receptors in the quadriceps muscle.
c True See above.
d True Impulses from the afferent neurones pass directly to the lower motor neurones of the quadriceps muscle.
e True Anaesthesia depresses all reflex activity. *(Ch. 5, A & S)*

60   Myocardial contractility is affected by

a   Heart rate.

b   Circulating volume.

c   Resting length of His-Purkinje fibres.

d   Parasympathetic activity.

e   Calcium.

61   A bellows spirometer (e.g. Vitalograph) may be used to measure

a   Expiratory reserve volume.

b   Closing volume.

c   Total lung capacity.

d   Functional residual capacity.

e   Residual volume.

62   Cerebral blood flow

a   Is reduced by hyperventilation.

b   Increases if arterial P_{O_2} is less than 7 kPa.

c   Remains stable over a mean arterial pressure range of 60–130 mmHg.

d   Increases with increased JVP.

e   Is dependent on intracranial pressure.

63   Ventilatory minute volume is increased by

a   Ascent to altitude.

b   A Pa_{O_2} of 10 kPa.

c   Chronic anaemia.

d   An Fi_{O_2} of 0.03.

e   Inspired CO_2 concentration of 0.03%.

a False Heart rate and contractility are usually independent.
b True The preload is determined partly by the circulating blood volume. An increased venous return to the heart increases end-diastolic fibre length, and thus myocardial contractility is increased (Frank-Starling relationship).
c False The His-Purkinje system is the 'electrical conducting' system of the heart, which transmits the wave of depolarisation from the atrioventricular node into the ventricles.
d True Vagal stimulation decreases contractility and also heart rate.
e True Calcium ions increase contractility.

---

a True The expiratory reserve volume is that volume which can be exhaled after a normal tidal volume. *(Appx. XI, A & S)*
b False Closing volume is measured usually by the nitrogen washout technique.
c False Total lung capacity includes residual volume and this cannot be measured using simple spirometry.
d False Functional residual capacity comprises expiratory reserve volume and residual volume. This is usually determined by means of a dilution technique using an indicator such as helium.
e False Residual volume cannot be measured by simple spirometry (*vide supra*).

---

a True Hypocapnia results in a reduction in cerebral blood flow.
b True Hypoxaemia causes a dramatic increase in cerebral blood flow.
c True This is the usual autoregulatory range in a normotensive patient.

d False Increased jugular venous pressure may reduce cerebral perfusion pressure and thus cerebral blood flow.
e True

---

a True A reduction in P_{IO_2} leads to a reduction in Pa_{O_2} with stimulation of peripheral chemoreceptors.
b False A Pa_{O_2} of 10 kPa represents the lower limit of the normal range for a healthy individual.
c False With chronic anaemia, there is no increase in ventilatory minute volume. However, 2, 3-DPG concentration increases and this enhances oxygen carrying capacity.
d True An F_{IO_2} of 0.03 increases ventilatory minute volume transiently, prior to death from hypoxaemia.
e False This is the normal concentration of carbon dioxide in the atmosphere.

64 **The oxyhaemoglobin dissociation curve is shifted to the right by**

a   Raised Pa_{CO_2}.

b   Raised 2,3-DPG.

c   Hypokalaemia.
d   Hypothermia.
e   Fetal haemoglobin.

65 **The following are anterior pituitary hormones**

a   FSH.

b   Arginine vasopressin.

c   Prolactin.

d   Corticotrophin releasing hormone.
e   Erythropoietin.

66 **Bilirubin**

a   Contains products of cytochrome metabolism.

b   When unconjugated, is bound to globulin in the plasma.
c   Is excreted in the bile mostly as the monoglucuronide.
d   Appears in excess concentration in the blood in its conjugated form in hepatic disease.
e   Is not detectable in the urine of healthy patients in its conjugated form.

67 **The liver is the major metabolic site of the following**

a   Insulin.
b   Glucagon.
c   Oestrogens.
d   Thyroxine.
e   Lignocaine.

(Ch. 2, A & S)

a True Carbon dioxide and hydrogen ions shift the curve to the right, thus facilitating oxygen unloading.

b True At a constant hydrogen ion concentration, increased 2, 3-DPG concentration decreases the affinity of haemoglobin for oxygen.

c False

d False Hypothermia shifts the curve to the left.

e False The oxyhaemoglobin dissociation curve of fetal haemoglobin has a P_{50} which is lower than that of adult haemoglobin.

(Ch. 12, D)

a True Follicle stimulating hormone (FSH) is released from the anterior pituitary.

b False Arginine vasopressin (ADH) is secreted by the neurohypophysis (posterior lobe).

c True Prolactin is under the inhibitory control of dopamine which is secreted by the hypothalamus.

d False This is secreted by the hypothalamus.

e False This is secreted by the kidney. (Ch. 13, D)

(Ch. 10, D)

a True 20% of bilirubin comprises products of catabolism of enzymes such as cytochromes and peroxidases.

b False Unconjugated bilirubin is bound to albumin.

c False 80% of bilirubin in bile is the diglucuronide.

d True Serum bilirubin follows the progress of hepatic disease and its treatment.

e True

(Ch. 10, D)

a True

b True

c True

d False Thyroxine undergoes widespread tissue metabolism.

e True The liver is the main site of drug metabolism.

68   Cardiac output in a normal subject

a   Increases with increased CVP.
b   Increases with increases in metabolic rate.
c   Increases in pyrexia.
d   Increases with increase in systemic arterial pressure.

e   Decreases with raised pulmonary capillary wedge pressure (PCWP).

69   Impulse propagation in a nerve

a   Is faster in non-myelinated nerves.

b   Occurs as a result of ionic transfer across the membrane.
c   Occurs as a result of electrical activity across the membrane.
d   May occur at 120 m/s.
e   May be slowed by prilocaine.

70   Oxygen

a   May cause convulsions at hyperbaric pressure.

b   Forms an inflammable mixture with air.
c   Is manufactured by fractional distillation of air.
d   Has a critical temperature of 36.5°C.

e   Causes bone marrow depression with prolonged administration.

71   Hyperventilation occurs in response to

a   Metabolic acidosis.
b   High altitude.

c   Low CSF pH.
d   Increase in base excess.

e   Deep sleep.

(Ch. 3, A & S)

a True This is induced by the Frank-Starling mechanism.
b True This is a normal physiological response.
c True
d False Cardiac output and peripheral resistance together determine systemic arterial pressure.
e False Cardiac output increases with increased PCWP.

(Ch. 5, A & S)

a False Myelinated nerves conduct faster than unmyelinated fibres (120 m/s: 0.5–2 m/s).
b True This is the process of depolarisation.
c False Electrical charges reflect ionic shifts but do not cause them.
d True See above.
e True Local anaesthetic agents block the Na^+/K^+ conduction channels.
(Ch. 15, A & S)

(Ch. 9, A & S)

a True Convulsions may occur with 100% O_2 at a pressure exceeding 2 atmospheres.
b False Although oxygen supports combustion, it is not itself flammable.
c True The other major product of this process is nitrogen.
d False The critical temperature of oxygen is -119°C; that of nitrous oxide is 36.5°C.
e False Nitrous oxide causes bone marrow depression after prolonged use.

(Ch. 2, A & S)

a True
b True At high altitude, the reduction in F_{IO_2} leads to hypoxaemia; unacclimatised subjects respond to this by hyperventilation.
c True This stimulates the central chemoreceptors.
d False An increase in base excess accompanies alkalosis or decreased hydrogen ion concentration. *(Ch. 22, A & S)*
e False The normal response to deep sleep is hypoventilation. Sleep apnoea syndrome represents a severe form of this.

72   The liver

  a   Receives its blood supply predominantly from the hepatic artery.
  b   Has a blood supply controlled by an autoregulatory mechanism.

  c   Is palpable normally below the right costal margin.

  d   Contains large stores of vitamin K.

  e   Undergoes shrinkage with advancing age and cirrhosis.

---

73   In a well-oxygenated, otherwise healthy middle-aged man, a Pa_{CO_2} of 6.1 kPa causes

  a   Pulmonary vasoconstriction.

  b   Cerebral vasodilatation.
  c   Release of catecholamines.

  d   Raised systemic arterial pressure.

  e   Low urinary pH.

---

74   The following are true of albumin

  a   It has a molecular weight of 70 000 daltons.

  b   Its plasma concentration is usually 35-50 g/litre.

  c   Hyperalbuminaemia occurs in liver failure.
  d   It has an important transport role.

  e   It is excreted in excess in nephrotic syndrome.

---

75   In the peripheral blood

  a   Normally, about 3% of total oxygen content is carried as dissolved oxygen.
  b Pa_{O_2} is normally the same as PA_{O_2}.

  c   Arterial P_{CO_2} is determined solely by the minute ventilation.

  d   Carbon dioxide is transported largely as bicarbonate.

  e   Whilst breathing air, the partial pressure of nitrogen is unchanged between arterial and venous blood.

(Ch. 10, D)

a False The portal vein supplies approximately 60% of liver blood flow.
b True Hepatic arterial flow may compensate for variations in portal venous flow.
c True Normally, there is descent of the liver on inspiration and the liver is palpable on deep inspiration.
d False Storage capacity for vitamin K is small, in contrast to that for vitamins D and B_{12}.
e True Liver reserve is reduced in the elderly and in later stages of cirrhosis.

(Ch. 8, D)

a False Pulmonary vasoconstriction is usually mediated via hypoxaemia. (Ch. 39, A & S)
b True
c True The sweaty, flushed appearance of hypercapnic patients is caused by release of catecholamines.
d True Catecholamine release causes an increase in systemic arterial pressure.
e True The kidneys compensate for a respiratory acidosis by excreting acid. (Ch. 22, A & S)

---

a True The average molecular weight of albumin is approximately 70 000 daltons. (Ch. 4, A & S)
b True This is the normal plasma concentration of albumin. (Appx. III, A & S)
c False Liver failure is characterised by hypoalbuminaemia. (Ch. 10, D)
d True Many drugs undergo protein binding which facilitates rapid distribution in vivo (Ch. 8, A & S)
e True Hypoproteinaemic oedema occurs in nephrotic syndrome secondary to albumin loss. (Ch. 11, D)

(Ch. 2, A & S)

a False Approximately 1.5% of oxygen content of arterial blood is dissolved in plasma normally.
b False There is a normally a small alveolar-arterial partial pressure difference because of the presence of physiological shunting and V/Q scatter.
c False Arterial P_{CO_2} is determined by CO_2 production and minute ventilation.
d True Carbonic acid dissociation in the red blood cell liberates bicarbonate ions which diffuse into the plasma.
e True Tissues do not produce nitrogen.

76   With respect to the control of ventilation

a   The chemoreceptors in the carotid and aortic bodies are stimulated by anaemia.

b   Marked respiratory stimulation occurs when F_{IO_2} < 60 mmHg.

c   Hypoxaemia increases the ventilatory response to hypercapnia.

d   When Pa_{CO_2} chronically exceeds Pa_{O_2} the respiratory centre is depressed by hypercapnia.

e   Afferents from the carotid bodies ascend to the medulla via the vagus nerve.

77   Effects of hypercapnia include

a   Coma when Pa_{CO_2} exceeds 10 kPa.

b   A reduction in sympathetic tone.

c   An increase in serum potassium concentration.

d   An increase in CSF pressure.

e   Potentiation of depolarising relaxants.

78   Central venous pressure

a   Always represents left atrial pressure.

b   Decreases with the onset of tachycardia in the healthy young patient.

c   Increases with fluid overload.

d   May be 5 mmHg in the normal individual.

e   May be measured in the inferior vena cava.

79   The following are neurotransmitters at autonomic ganglia

a   Adrenaline.

b   Noradrenaline.

c   Dopamine.

d   5-Hydroxytryptamine (5-HT).

e   Acetylcholine.

(Ch. 2, A & S)

a False Peripheral chemoreceptors respond to Pa_{O_2} and not oxygen content or haemoglobin concentration.

b False Respiratory stimulation occurs when Pa_{O_2} is less than 60 mmHg (8 kPa). FI_{O_2} is the inspired *fractional* concentration of oxygen.

c True The slope of the carbon dioxide response curve is increased in the presence of hypoxaemia.

d True Care should be exercised during administration of postoperative oxygen therapy.

e False The carotid sinus nerve is a branch of the glossopharyngeal nerve.

(Ch. 8, D)

a True Drowsiness and coma supervene with severe hypercapnia.

b False Hypercapnia stimulates the sympathetic nervous system and cardiac output is increased.

c True Hypercapnia leads to acidosis and favours movement of intracellular potassium into the extracellular fluid. *(Ch. 22, A & S)*

d True Carbon dioxide is a potent vasodilator.

e False There is no potentiation of neuromuscular block.

(Ch. 3, A & S)

a False Central venous pressure reflects right atrial pressure. It reflects left atrial pressure only in the absence of pulmonary hypertension, mitral valve disease, etc; in these situations, pulmonary capillary wedge pressure is a better indicator of left atrial pressure.

b True There is a transient decrease in central venous pressure with the onset of tachycardia.

c True This is an early sign of fluid overload.

d True The normal range for central venous pressure is 0–7 mmHg. *(Appx. IV, A & S)*

e True Provided that the end of the measuring catheter is intrathoracic.

(Ch. 5, A & S)

a False

b False Noradrenaline is the postganglionic neurotransmitter in most of the sympathetic nervous system.

c False Dopamine is a neurotransmitter at central sites but not at peripheral ganglia.

d False 5-HT is a central neurotransmitter found in the brain stem and spinal cord.

e True

80   The following changes tend to occur postoperatively

    a Hypoglycaemia.

    b Decreased K^+ excretion.

    c Increased production of cortisol.

    d Increased production of adrenaline.

    e Raised serum concentration of antidiuretic hormone (ADH).

81   In respect of the ABO blood groups

    a These are inherited in Mendelian fashion.
    b A patient with group AB has anti-A and anti-B antibodies.
    c Antibodies are found in saliva.
    d Blood may be typed independently if anti-A and anti-B serum is available.
    e Group AB is the universal recipient.

82   Increased vagal activity results in

    a Reduced rate of depolarisation of the cardiac muscle.
    b Reduced SA nodal activity.
    c Reduced AV nodal activity.
    d Raised threshold potential.
    e Changes in potassium permeability.

83   The following factors increase production of renin

    a Reduction in renal perfusion pressure.

    b Increased intracellular $[Na^+]$ and decreased extracellular $[K^+]$.

    c Angiotensin II.

    d Decreased plasma volume.

    e Lumbar extradural block.

a False The sympatho-adrenal response to surgery and stress involves mobilisation of glucose via gluconeogenesis and glycogenolysis.
b False Increased secretion of cortisol and aldosterone results in sodium and water retention and potassium excretion.
c True This is part of the endocrine response to stress and surgery. Steroid-treated patients must receive perioperative replacement therapy. *(Ch. 41, A & S)*
d True Increased sympatho-adrenal activity is part of the stress response to surgery.
e True Antidiuretic hormone is secreted in response to stress, augmenting the water retention which occurs postoperatively. *(Ch. 12, D)*

(Ch. 7, A & S)

a True In the United Kingdom, 47% of persons are group O.
b False Group AB has neither anti-A nor anti-B antibodies in the serum.
c True Antibodies in saliva give an indication of the ABO blood group.
d True This is the basis of blood grouping tests.

e True Group AB has no serum antibodies.

(Ch. 3, A & S)

a True
b True
c False There is no vagal innervation of the AV node.
d False The threshold potential of -50 mV is unaffected.
e False Changes in potassium permeability affect the resting membrane potential. This is unaffected by vagal activity.

(Ch. 4, A & S)

a True A baroreceptor mechanism in the afferent arteriole detects a decrease in renal blood flow.
b False Increased secretion of renin and aldosterone is caused by a decrease in extracellular sodium concentration or increased extracellular potassium concentration.
c False Angiotensin II is part of the pathway between renin and the stimulation of aldosterone secretion. Angiotensin II suppresses secretion of renin.
d True A reduction in plasma volume results in reduction in renal perfusion pressure.
e True Sympathetic block results in hypotension and decreased renal perfusion pressure.

84 **The following values for water distribution are correct for a 70 kg man**

    a Total body water (TBW) = 49 litre.

    b Intracellular fuid (ICF) = 28 litre.

    c Extracellular fluid (ECF) = 21 litre.

    d Plasma volume = 3.5 litre.

    e Interstitial fluid = 3.5 litre.

85 **ADH production**

    a Is stimulated by morphine and ether.

    b Is under hypothalamic control.

    c Is stimulated by increase in plasma osmolality.

    d Is inhibited by decrease in plasma volume.

    e Is inhibited by ethanol.

86 **The following may cause sodium retention**

    a Congestive cardiac failure.

    b Hepatic failure.

    c Infusion of hypotonic fluid.

    d Excessive sweating.

    e Oedema.

87 **Pulmonary function tests in a 25-year-old female of 58 kg reveal FEV_1 2.45 litre; FVC 3.0 litre. These may indicate**

    a A diagnosis of asthma.

    b The patient is asymptomatic.

    c The need for an urgent ventilation/perfusion scan.

    d Myasthenia gravis.

    e Hyperventilation.

(Appx. VI, Ch. 4, A & S)

a False Total body water is 60% of body weight which would be 42 litre in a 70 kg man.
b True Intracellular fluid volume is two-thirds of the total body water.
c False Extracellular fluid volume would amount to 14 litre.
d True Plasma volume is 50 ml/kg in an adult.
e False Interstitial fluid volume is ECF minus plasma volume, i.e. approximately 10.5 litre.

(Ch. 5, D)

a True ADH (vasopressin) release may be stimulated by drugs such as morphine, phenothiazines, and tricyclic antidepressants. Ether has sympathomimetic actions and may stimulate ADH.
b True Osmoreceptors are situated in the hypothalamus. *(Ch. 4, A & S)*
c True An increase in plasma osmolality stimulates the synthesis of ADH in the supra-optic nuclei.
d False A 15% decrease in plasma volume with no change in osmolality stimulates secretion of ADH. *(Ch. 12, D)*.
e True This accounts for the diuretic effect of alcohol.

a True Secondary hyperaldosteronism occurs, resulting in sodium retention. *(Ch. 12, D)*
b True In hepatic failure, hormone metabolism is impaired and the actions of aldosterone are prolonged *(Ch. 10, D)*
c False After infusion of a hypotonic fluid, some sodium is excreted with the excess water.
d False Excess sweat contains little sodium and does not alter sodium homeostasis significantly. *(Appx., D)*
e True Oedema is frequently associated with sodium retention. *(Ch. 5, D)*

(Ch. 8, D; Appx. XI, A & S)

a False The FEV_1/FVC ratio is normal (approximately 80%). In asthma, this ratio is reduced.
b True These values are normal for a 25-year-old of short stature.
c False See **b**.
d True These values may be found in a well-controlled myasthenic. However, both FEV_1 and FVC may be reduced greatly in an undiagnosed or poorly controlled myasthenic patient. *(Ch. 41, A & S)*
e False Pulmonary function tests do not give any indication of ventilatory rate or tidal volume.

88   Ingestion of 20 ml/kg water over a period of 20 min normally results in

a   Increased urine output for 12 h.

b   Reduction in interstitial fluid osmolality.

c   Increased secretion of ADH.

d   Stimulation of carotid sinus receptors.

e   Increase in atrial natriuretic hormone production.

89   In the full term neonate

a   Pulmonary arterial pressure declines in the first two weeks.

b   The oxyhaemoglobin dissociation curve is shifted to the right.
c   Unconjugated jaundice is common during the first week.

d   Approximately 80% of haemoglobin is HbF.

e   Vitamin K should be administered to counteract the development of jaundice.

90   In the renal tubule

a   Almost 95% of the glomerular filtrate is reabsorbed.
b   65% of sodium is absorbed in the proximal convoluted tubule (PCT).
c   Aldosterone increases sodium absorption in the PCT.

d   Hydrogen ions are excreted mostly as phosphate.

e   Arginine vasopressin increases water permeability in the collecting ducts.

(Ch. 22, A & S; Ch. 5, D)

a False The increased urine output resulting from ingestion of 1.4 litre in a 70 kg man would last for approximately 1–2 h.

b True This water load would lead to a reduction in interstitial fluid osmolality.

c False ADH secretion would be increased in the presence of dehydration or increased interstitial fluid osmolality.

d False The carotid sinus receptors respond to increased arterial pressure. Changes in plasma volume are sensed by atrial (predominantly right) volume receptors.

e True Stimulation of the atrial stretch receptors increases production of atrial natriuretic hormone. *(Ch. 4, A & S)*

(Ch. 6, A & S)

a True There is a rapid decline from fetal values at first, then a gradual reduction to reach adult values after two weeks.

b False The presence of HbF shifts the curve to the left.

c True This is more likely in the presence of hypoglycaemia and hypothermia, and is treated by phototherapy.

d True The subsequent decline in production of HbF with conversion to synthesis of HbA contributes to the physiological anaemia of infancy.

e False Vitamin K is given to supplement the neonatal hepatic stores and promote synthesis of coagulation factors.

(Ch. 4, A & S; Ch. 11, D)

a False Approximately 99% of glomerular filtrate is reabsorbed.

b True Active transport in combination with passive transport accounts for absorption of the majority of filtered sodium at this site.

c False Aldosterone increases sodium absorption in the distal convoluted tubule and the collecting duct.

d False Hydrogen ions are excreted in combination with ammonia (67%) and phosphate (33%).

e True Arginine vasopressin is ADH and is secreted in response to increased extracellular fluid osmolality.

91   Cardiac output

a   Is the product of heart rate and systemic vascular resistance.

b   May be measured by the Fick principle.

c   May be measured by a technique involving 5% glucose.

d   Increase is always accompanied by increased oxygen consumption.

e   Is reduced more by isoflurane than by halothane.

92   The first rib

a   Is grooved by the subclavian vein.

b   Articulates with the body of the sternum.

c   Is the insertion for scalenus anterior.

d   Is crossed by the cords of the brachial plexus.

e   Forms part of the thoracic inlet.

93   In the normal cardiac cycle

a   The right ventricle contracts before the left.

b   The right atrium contracts before the left atrium.

c   The interventricular septum depolarises from left to right.

d   The normal PR interval is 0.22 s.

e   The refractory period of cardiac muscle is 0.5 s.

94   Coagulation of blood

a   Initially involves the aggregation of platelets at the point of vessel damage.

b   Involves the production of thrombin from factor II.

c   Occurs under the influence of either an intrinsic system or an extrinsic cascade.

d   Is impaired in haemophilia B as a result of deficiency of factor IX.

e   Is inhibited by activation of antithrombin III by heparin.

(Ch. 3, A & S)

a False Cardiac output is the product of heart rate and stroke volume.
b True This is the standard method of measurement; cardiac output is equal to oxygen consumption divided by the arterio-venous oxygen content difference.
c True In the thermodilution technique, cold glucose is injected into the right atrium and temperature change measured in the pulmonary artery.
d False Increases in cardiac output may occur without an increase in oxygen consumption.
e False Halothane reduces myocardial contractility to a greater extent than does isoflurane. *(Ch. 9, A & S)*

(Ch. 1, Ch. 26, A & S)

a True The vein runs anterior to the artery and brachial plexus.
b False The first rib articulates with the manubrium sterni.
c True The scalenus anterior muscle is inserted between the subclavian artery and vein.
d False The cords of the brachial plexus surround the axillary artery. The roots of the brachial plexus lie behind the scalenus anterior and the trunks emerge from its lateral border.
e True Together with T1 and the manubrium sterni.

(Ch. 3, A & S)

a False The right atrium contracts before the left atrium but the ventricles normally contract synchronously.
b True See above.
c True The bundle of His supplying the left ventricle depolarises first. This leads to the initial Q wave of a ventricular depolarisation.
d False The normal PR interval is 0.12–0.2 s. An interval of 0.22 s indicates first degree heart block. *(Appx. IV, A & S)*
e False The refractory period is normally less than 0.3 s.

(Ch. 7, A & S; Ch. 13, D)

a False The initial action is vessel spasm and platelet adhesion.
b True Prothrombin (factor II) is converted to thrombin under the influence of activated factor X.
c True The intrinsic system is more potent. Both systems result in activation of factor X.
d True Factor IX (Christmas factor) deficiency leads to a similar clinical picture to classical haemophilia.
e False Antithrombin III is a naturally occurring thrombin inactivator which is potentiated by heparin.

95   Intraocular pressure (IOP) is

    a   Less than atmospheric when the globe is open.

    b   Decreased by halothane.

    c   Decreased by a 15° head-up tilt.

    d   Increased throughout the duration of a Valsalva manoeuvre.

    e   Increased by hypercapnia.

96   Dilatation of the blood vessels in the skin of the left hand may be caused by

    a   Halothane.

    b   Cyclopropane.

    c   Immersing the right hand in hot water.

    d   Drinking 500 ml of warm milk.
    e   Hyperventilation.

97   In the normal lungs

    a   Inspiration of 100% O_2 may dilate pulmonary blood vessels.

    b   Ventilation is greater at the apex of the lung.
    c   5-Hydroxytryptamine causes an increase in bronchial resistance.
    d   Histamine increases the pulmonary arterial pressure.

    e   Noradrenaline increases pulmonary vascular resistance.

98   The following are used in indicator dilution methods to measure cardiac output

    a   Indocyanine green.

    b   Fick principle.

    c   Cuvette densitometer.

    d   Interferometer.

    e   Polarography.

(Ch. 29, A & S)

a False When the globe is opened, intraocular pressure becomes the same as atmospheric pressure.

b True Halothane, in common with other volatile anaesthetic agents, decreases intraocular pressure.

c True Intraocular pressure is dependent upon central venous pressure which is reduced by a 15° head-up tilt.

d False Although there is a transient increase in intraocular pressure with increased intrathoracic pressure, the adaptive mechanism counteracts any sustained rise.

e True There is a linear relationship between intraocular pressure and arterial carbon dioxide tension.

(Ch. 9, A & S)

a True Peripheral vasodilatation is a feature of spontaneous ventilation with halothane. If Pa_{CO_2} is controlled, halothane has no effect.

b True Cyclopropane causes respiratory depression and hypercapnia during spontaneous ventilation.

c True There is a direct and consensual component to vasodilatation with hot water immersion.

d True Although the effect may be transient!

e False Hyperventilation is associated with peripheral vasoconstriction as a result of hypocapnia.

(Ch. 2, A & S)

a True Hypoxic pulmonary vasoconstriction is abolished by inspiration of 100% oxygen. *(Ch. 39, A & S)*

b False Ventilation per unit volume is 50% greater at the base of the lung.

c True 5-Hydroxytryptamine causes bronchoconstriction. *(Ch. 36, A & S)*

d True Histamine produces pulmonary vasoconstriction but peripheral vasodilatation.

e True Noradrenaline causes pulmonary vasoconstriction.

(Ch. 3, A & S)

a True Indocyanine green is the indicator used normally in dye dilution methods.

b False This may be used to measure cardiac output but is not the principle underlying indicator dilution methods.

c True The Cuvette densitometer is used in the measurement of indocyanine green concentration; sampling is usually from the radial artery.

d False An interferometer is used to measure gas concentration, e.g. in the calibration of vaporisers.

e False Polarography is a method of measuring oxygen concentration.

99 **The following may prolong gastric emptying**

    a   Atropine.

    b   Metoclopramide.

    c   Morphine.

    d   Cimetidine.

    e   Nalbuphine.

---

100 **In respect of the cardiovascular system during pregnancy**

    a   Cardiac output increases in the first trimester.

    b   Peripheral resistance is unaltered.

    c   Venous return is obstructed in the supine position after the 13th week.

    d   Pulmonary vascularity is increased on chest X-ray.

    e   Circulation time is decreased.

(Ch. 4, BNF)

a **True**
b **False** Metoclopramide increases gastric motility. *(Ch. 14, A & S)*
c **True** Morphine reduces gastrointestinal motility and delays gastric emptying in particular. *(Ch. 11, A & S)*
d **False** Cimetidine has no effect on gastric emptying or gastrointestinal motility.
e **True** Nalbuphine is an opioid analgesic and delays gastric emptying.

(Ch. 6, A & S)

a **True** Contractility, heart rate and stroke volume increase, resulting in an increase of approximately 1.5 litre/min.
b **False** Peripheral resistance decreases in mid-trimester because of new vessel formation and reduced vascular tone.
c **True** The supine hypotensive syndrome may occur after the beginning of the second trimester.
d **True** Pulmonary blood flow is increased and this is evident as increased vascularity in the chest X-ray.
e **False** There is no significant change in circulation time.

2. Pharmacology

1   **A highly ionised drug**

   a   Is well absorbed from the intestine.

   b   Is excreted mainly in the kidney.

   c   Crosses the placenta easily.
   d   Is reabsorbed from the renal tubule.

   e   Is highly protein bound.

2   **Sodium nitroprusside decreases arterial pressure by**

   a   An action on alpha-receptors.

   b   Reducing cardiac output.

   c   Causing bradycardia.

   d   Producing cyanide ions.

   e   A direct action on blood vessels.

3   **The following are eliminated by the kidney mainly in the unchanged form:**

   a   Vecuronium.

   b   Suxamethonium.

   c   Dopamine.
   d   Gallamine.

   e   Digoxin.

(Ch. 8, A & S)

a False The undissociated moiety of a drug crosses membranes in the gastrointestinal tract. Highly ionised drugs are less well absorbed.
b True Highly ionised drugs are water soluble and are excreted readily by the kidney.
c False Drugs in the ionised form are poorly lipid soluble.
d False The pKa and acidity of the filtrate determine the extent of ionisation within the renal tubules, but in general terms, ionised drugs are reabsorbed poorly at this site.
e False Highly lipid soluble drugs undergo protein binding to a greater extent than ionised drugs, which are freely soluble in plasma.

(Ch. 37, A & S)

a False Sodium nitroprusside is a direct acting vasodilator and does not act via adrenoceptors.
b False Nitroprusside affects predominantly resistance vessels and has no direct effect on cardiac contractility.
c False Hypotension induced by nitroprusside is accompanied by reflex tachycardia.
d False Nitroprusside is metabolised to cyanide ions, which may reach toxic concentrations after prolonged administration. However, this is not related to its hypotensive action.
e True

a False Vecuronium is metabolised by the liver and excreted in the bile.
(Ch. 12, A & S)
b False Suxamethonium undergoes ester hydrolysis by plasma cholinesterases *(Ch. 12, A & S)*
c False Dopamine is metabolised extensively throughout the body.
d True Gallamine is excreted almost entirely by the kidney; administration is contraindicated in patients with renal impairment. *(Ch. 12, A & S)*
e True Digoxin should be administered with reduced frequency in the presence of renal impairment. *(Ch. 14, A & S)*

4   Edrophonium is used for

a   Testing for the presence of myasthenia gravis.
b   Antagonism of neuromuscular blockade.

c   Producing central respiratory stimulation.
d   Relief of urinary retention.

e   Treatment of myotonia congenita.

5   Morphine administered extradurally

a   May cause intense itching.
b   May cause urinary retention.
c   May produce nausea and vomiting.

d   Leads to delayed respiratory depression not relieved by
    naloxone.
e   Acts by binding to receptors in the postcentral gyrus.

**6   An untoward reaction to the following may occur in a patient taking
        monoamine oxidase inhibitors**

a   Adrenaline.

b   Thiopentone.
c   Diazepam.
d   Tricyclic antidepressants.

e   Amphetamine.

7   Nitrous oxide

a   Increases cardiac output
b   Decreases peripheral resistance.

c   Causes no significant change in arterial blood pressure in healthy
    individuals.
d   Increases heart rate.
e   Sensitises the heart to exogenous catecholamines.

a True   This is described as the Tensilon test *(Ch. 15, D)*
b True   Edrophonium is an anticholinesterase and may be used for this purpose. *(Ch. 12, A & S)*
c False   Edrophonium does not possess respiratory stimulant properties.
d False   An anticholinesterase may be effective in relieving urinary retention. However, edrophonium is not used commonly for this purpose.
e False   It is not used for the treatment of this condition.

(Ch. 11, A & S)

a True   This is a commonly reported side-effect.
b True   Urinary retention is a common side-effect.
c True   Nausea and vomiting occur as frequently as with other routes of administration.
d False   Naloxone antagonises respiratory depression associated with extradural morphine.
e False   Spinal opioid receptors are located in the substantia gelatinosa *(Ch. 5, A & S)*

(Ch. 30, A & S)

a True   Augmentation of the action of adrenaline and other sympathomimetics occurs in the presence of MAOI drugs.
b False   Thiopentone has no sympathomimetic activity.
c False   Diazepam has no sympathomimetic activity.
d False   However the combination of tricyclic and MAOI antidepressants shoud be used with extreme caution.
e True   Amphetamine is a sympathomimetic agent; hypertensive crisis may occur with the combination. (Appx. 1 BNF)

(Ch. 9, A & S)

a False   Cardiac output is depressed.
b False   Peripheral resistance is increased; in combination with **a**, there is little change in arterial pressure in healthy individuals.
c True   See **b**.

d False   There is little effect on heart rate.
e False   This is true of halothane but not nitrous oxide.

8 Halothane

a Increases GI tract motility.

b Increases cerebral blood flow.
c Is metabolised to an extent of 10% of the administered dose.
d Increases cerebral metabolic rate.
e Increases intraocular pressure.

9 Enflurane

a Is an ether.

b Is inflammable but not explosive in concentrations greater than 4% in oxygen.
c Has the formula: $CHBrClCF_3$
d Is metabolised to yield free bromide ions.
e Is metabolised to yield free fluoride ions.

10 Ketamine

a Has antanalgesic properties.
b Is an antisialagogue.

c Increases heart rate.
d Must be given intramuscularly.
e May cause unpleasant dreams in children.

11 Depolarising neuromuscular block is associated with

a Fasciculations.
b Fade on tetanic stimulation.
c Enhancement by volatile agents.
d Antagonism by anticholinesterase drugs.
e Postoperative myalgia.

12 Factors which determine the rate of increase of alveolar concentration of a volatile agent include

a The biotransformation of the agent.
b Minute ventilation.

c The MAC of the agent.
d The inspired concentration of the agent.

e Cardiac output.

(Ch. 9, Ch. 38, A & S)

a False GI motility is depressed in common with the effect of other volatile agents.
b True Halothane causes cerebral vasodilatation.
c False 20% of an administered dose undergoes hepatic metabolism.
d False Cerebral metabolic rate is decreased.
e False Intraocular pressure is decreased.

(Ch. 9, A & S)

a True Enflurane is 2 chloro–1, 1, 2–trifluoethyl-difluoromethyl ether.
(Appx. II, A & S)
b False Enflurane is flammable at concentrations greater than 6% in oxygen.

c False This is halothane. (See **a**).
d False Enflurane contains no bromine.
e True Free fluoride is produced but not in sufficient concentration to cause renal damage.

(Ch. 10, A & S)

a False It has analgesic properties at subanaesthetic concentrations.
b False It may cause intense salivation, and premedication with atropine is recommended.
c True Heart rate is increased by facilitation of calcium transport.
d False It may be given intravenously.
e True But children complain less than do adults.

(Ch. 12, A & S)

a True This is a characteristic of depolarising block.
b False This is a characteristic of non-depolarising block.
c False This is a characteristic of non-depolarising block.
d False Anticholinesterases may prolong the block.
e True This is more prevalent in young ambulant patients.

(Ch. 8, A & S)

a False Biotransformation has virtually no influence.
b True The rate of increase is determined by the balance between input to, and uptake from, the lungs. For a given inspired concentration, an increase in minute ventilation increases rate of input.
c False MAC has no influence; it is a measure of potency.
d True Increasing the inspired concentration increases alveolar concentration for a given minute volume.
e True The relationship is inverse.

13 Lignocaine

a May be used for treatment of ventricular arrhythmias.

b Is used for epidural analgesia in a 4% solution.

c May cause methaemoglobinaemia.
d Should be used with special care in patients taking propranolol.

e Was first used for intravenous regional analgesia in 1908 by Augustus Bier.

14 Suxamethonium

a Acts as an antagonist at the neuromuscular junction.
b Is metabolised by hydrolysis.
c Hyperpolarises the transmembrane potential at the neuromuscular junction.
d Acts by increasing the flux of sodium and potassium ions.
e Antagonises tubocurarine.

15 Atropine

a Completely blocks the vagus nerve in a dose of 0.4 mg / 70 kg.
b May cause bradycardia in very low dose.
c Increases physiological dead space.
d Produces moderate CNS depression.
e Causes pupillary constriction.

16 Isoprenaline

a Stimulates the baroreceptors, resulting in bradycardia.
b Produces transient bronchospasm.
c Is used in a dose of 1–20 µg/min in adults to produce a positive inotropic effect.
d May be used for treatment of complete heart block.
e May cause hypotension because of action at alpha-adrenoceptors.

(Ch. 15, A & S)

a True It possesses membrane stabilising properties (Class I anti-arryhthmic). *(Ch. 14, A & S)*
b False The maximum recommended dose (200 mg) would be reached with 5 ml of 4% solution.
c False Prilocaine possesses this side effect.
d True Reduction in maintenance therapy of anti-arrhythmics is recommended. *(Ch. 14, A & S)*
e False Lignocaine was synthesised first in 1948, Bier used procaine.

(Ch. 12, A & S)

a False Suxamethonium is an agonist and causes depolarising block.
b True Ester hydrolysis by plasma cholinesterase.
c False The membrane is depolarised not hyperpolarised.

d True This is how depolarisation occurs.
e True This represents interaction between a competitive antagonist (dTC) and a drug which depolarises the NMJ, i.e an agonist.

(Ch. 13, A & S)

a False A dose greater than this would be required.
b True This may occur on i.v. administration.
c True This is caused by vagal blockade and bronchodilation.
d False Atropine may produce CNS excitation.
e False Atropine is a mydriatic.

(Ch. 13, A & S)

a False Beta-stimulation causes tachycardia.
b False Beta-stimulation results in bronchodilation.
c True 0.02 to 0.40 µg/kg per minute is the recommended dose. (Appex IV, A & S)
d True This is one of the main indications for its use.
e False Isoprenaline has no alpha adrenoceptor activity; diastolic arterial pressure may be reduced because of beta-effects on muscle blood vessels (vasodilatation), but systolic pressure is increased by a positive inotropic action.

17 **Tricyclic antidepressants**

a Depress the formation of noradrenaline.
b May cause hypertension.

c May cause arrhythmias.

d May cause renal failure after prolonged administration.
e May produce sedation.

18 **Thiopentone**

a 2.5% in aqueous solution has a pH of approximately 11.
b Is metabolised only by the kidney.
c Is an oxybarbiturate.
d Is stable in solution for 24 hours.
e May be used in a 10% solution.

19 **The response to an agonist drug**

a Occurs as a result of its high affinity and high intrinsic activity.
b May be antagonised with no change in its receptor affinity.

c May be antagonised competitively by a drug with high intrinsic activity.
d Is maximal at low concentrations if it is a partial agonist.

e Is a pharmacodynamic property of the drug.

20 **The following drugs may be used i.v. in anaesthetic practice for induced hypotension**

a Hexamethonium

b Captopril.

c Sodium nitroprusside.
d Glyceryl trinitrate.

e Trimetaphan.

(Ch. 30, A & S)

a False Noradrenaline re-uptake is inhibited. *(Ch. 16, D)*
b True These drugs should be given with caution to patients with heart disease.
c True Because of anticholinergic and sympathomimetic effects, overdosage may result in serious and intractable arrhythmias.
d False This is not a recognised side-effect in therapeutic doses.
e True

(Ch. 10, A & S)

a True
b False Thiopentone undergoes hepatic metabolism.
c False It is a thiobarbiturate. Pentobarbitone is its oxy-analogue.
d True And probably longer, but its use after 24 hours is not recommended.
e True But only for rectal administration. Solutions stronger than 2.5% should never be used i.v because of the risk of tissue damage associated with extravascular leakage.

(Ch. 8, A & S)

a True An agent with high affinity but no intrinsic activity is an antagonist.
b True This is non-competitive antagonism. No increase in agonist concentration will overcome the antagonism.
c False An antagonist has affinity but no intrinsic activity.

d False A partial agonist is unable to produce a maximal response, even at high concentrations.

e True

(Ch. 37, A & S)

a True Hexamethonium is a sympathetic ganglion blocker but is no longer available in the UK.
b False Captopril is an angiotensin-converting enzyme inhibitor which has been used as oral pretreatment before hypotensive anaesthesia. *(Ch. 14, A & S)*
c True It is a vasodilator which acts directly on blood vessel walls.
d True Glyceryl trinitrate has direct actions predominantly on the venous side of the circulation. *(Ch. 14, A & S)*
e True Trimetaphan is a sympathetic ganglion blocker with a short duration of action.

21   **The following agents cross the blood/ brain barrier**
   a   Tubocurarine.
   b   Hexamethonium.
   c   Lignocaine.

   d   Hyoscine hydrobromide.

   e   Sulphadimidine.

22   **The following statements are true**
   a   Cimetidine potentiates the effects of warfarin.
   b   Erythromycin potentiates the effects of theophylline.
   c   Isoflurane potentiates the effects of pancuronium.
   d   Rifampicin potentiates the effects of glucocorticoids.

   e   Propranolol antagonises the effects of verapamil.

23   **Dopamine**
   a   Crosses the blood brain barrier.
   b   Is a precursor of L-dopa.

   c   Increases renal blood flow in low dose.

   d   Is ineffective orally.
   e   Causes coronary vasoconstriction.

24   **Etomidate**
   a   Is excreted unchanged by the kidneys.

   b   Is dissolved in propylene glycol.
   c   Decreases intraocular pressure.
   d   Causes more venous sequelae than thiopentone.

   e   Suppresses adrenocortical function.

a False   This is a polar molecule, and poorly lipid soluble. *(Ch. 12, A & S)*
b False   Hexamethonium, a ganglion blocker, is also a polar molecule.
c True   The undissociated form of lignocaine (free base) is lipid soluble and free to cross the blood/brain barrier. *(Ch. 15. A & S)*
d True   Hyoscine may cause central nervous system depression, especially in the elderly. *(Ch. 13, A & S)*
e True   Sulphonamides are effective in the treatment of meningococcal meningitis. *(Ch. 3, D)*

(Appx. 1, BNF)

a True
b True   This may result in theophylline toxicity
c True   *(Ch. 9, A & S)*
d True   Rifampicin is an anti-tuberculous drug which causes liver enzyme induction *(Ch. 8, D)*
e False   Verapamil is not recommended in combination with a beta-adrenergic blocker *(Ch. 7, D)*

(Ch. 13, A & S)

a False
b False   Tyrosine is oxidised to L-dopa and this is decarboxylated to dopamine. Dopamine is a precursor of noradrenaline and adrenaline.
c True   In a dose of up to 5 µg/kg per minute, the major effect of dopamine is on the renal vasculature.
d True   Dopamine is given by intravenous infusion.
e False   But in high doses (greater than 15 µg/kg per minute) peripheral vasoconstriction occurs.

(Ch. 10, A & S)

a True   Although a small proportion of etomidate is excreted unchanged, the majority is broken down rapidly by hydrolysis.
b True   It is dissolved in water with 35% propylene glycol at pH 8.1.
c True   This is true of all intravenous anaesthetic agents except ketamine.
d True   Pain on injection occurs in up to 80% of patients; this may be minimised by rapid injection into a large vein.
e True   By suppression of 11-beta-hydroxylase. *(Ch. 9, A & S)*

25 Which of the following are alpha-blockers?

a Phentolamine.
b Oxprenolol.
c Phenoxybenzamine.

d Labetalol.

e Prazosin.

26 Digoxin

a Causes bronchoconstriction.
b Decreases central venous pressure.
c Enhances appetite.
d Increases pulmonary artery pressure.
e Increases urine output.

27 Epileptiform activity may be seen after the following

a Propofol.

b Halothane.
c Bupivacaine.

d Enflurane.

e Hypoxaemia.

28 Dantrolene

a Is formulated in aqueous solution.
b May only be given i.v.

c Decreases release of calcium at the sarcoplasmic reticulum.

d Causes abnormal liver function tests.

e Does not affect the neuromuscular junction.

(Ch. 13, A & S)

a True Phentolamine is a short-acting alpha-adrenoceptor blocking drug.
b False Oxprenolol is a beta-adrenoceptor blocking drug.
c True Phenoxybenzamine is a relatively long-acting alpha-adrenoceptor blocking drug.
d True Labetalol is a combined alpha and beta-blocker with a relative activity of alpha: beta-blockade of 3:7.
e True Prazosin is a post-synaptic, alpha-blocking agent with vasodilator properties.

(Ch. 14, A & S)

a False
b True Secondary to positive inotropic effects.
c False Loss of appetite is a common feature.
d False Digoxin has no direct effect upon pulmonary vessels.
e True Secondary to improved cardiac output.

---

a True There have been reports of seizure activity associated with propofol, although it reduces duration of seizure during ECT. *(Ch. 10, A & S)*
b False *(Ch. 9, A & S)*
c True Toxic levels of bupivacaine may cause CNS depression and epileptiform activity. *(Ch. 15, A & S)*
d True Enflurane is associated with epileptiform activity on EEG if more than 3% has been administered; epileptic activity per se is not a recognised feature of enflurane anaesthesia.
e True This is a late sign of cerebral damage.

(Ch. 23, A & S; Ch. 15, BNF)

a False It is formulated in mannitol for i.v. administration.
b False It may be given orally preoperatively as prophylaxis in a patient with malignant hyperthermia susceptibility.
c True Dantrolene interferes with calcium efflux in the muscle cell, preventing the contractile process.
d True Liver function tests should be checked regularly in patients receiving long-term therapy.
e True Its site of action is on the sarcoplasmic reticulum.

29 Propranolol

a Has local anaesthetic effects.
b Causes postural hypotension.
c Is contraindicated in patients with paroxysmal nocturnal dyspnoea (PND) and orthopnoea.
d Has a half-life of 6 hours.
e Is a cardioselective beta-agonist.

30 Glyceryl trinitrate causes

a Reduction in pulmonary arterial pressure.

b Reduction in preload.
c Bronchospasm.
d Headache.
e Relief of angina as a result of coronary artery dilatation.

31 The following drugs are absorbed well from the alimentary tract

a Ergotamine.

b Oxytocin.
c Atropine.

d Pentamethonium.
e Adrenaline.

32 The opium poppy contains

a Diamorphine.
b Codeine.
c Papaverine.
d Methadone.
e Strophanthin.

(Ch. 13, A & S)

a **True** This is not a characteristic of all beta-blocking agents.
b **False**
c **True** Orthopnoea and PND indicate incipient heart failure which is an absolute contraindication to propranolol therapy.
d **False** The majority of beta-blockers have a half-life of 3–4 hours.
e **False** Propranolol is neither cardioselective nor an agonist.

(Ch. 14, A & S)

a **True** It is predominantly a venodilator, but also causes pulmonary vasodilatation.
b **True** Venodilatation leads to a reduction in CVP and preload.
c **False**
d **True** This is a common side-effect because of cerebral vasodilatation.
e **False** Reduction in preload leads to reduction in myocardial oxygen consumption. (Ch.7, D)

a **False** This drug is frequently given orally, but absorption is unpredictable and the recommended routes of administration are sublingual, rectal or by inhalation. (Ch. 15, D)
b **False** This is usually given intravenously or by nasal spray. (Ch. 7, BNF)
c **True** This has antispasmodic actions and is available as oral tablets. (Ch. 1, BNF)
d **False** Pentamethonium is a highly polar compound.
e **False** Adrenaline is degraded by the intestinal mucosa and by first-pass metabolism in the liver. (Ch. 3, BNF)

(Ch. 11, A & S)

a **False** Diamorphine (di-acetylmorphine) is a semi-synthetic drug.
b **True**
c **True**
d **False** Methadone is a synthetic opioid.
e **False** Strophanthin is an alternative name for ouabain, a cardiac glycoside. (Ch. 14, A & S)

33   The following antimicrobials are active against Gram-negative bacilli

a   Nitrofurantoin.

b   Erythromycin.

c   Benzylpenicillin.
d   Mecillinam.

e   Chloramphenicol.

34   The following are side-effects of sulphonamides

a   Nephrotic syndrome.

b   VIIIth nerve damage.

c   Crystalluria.
d   Haemolytic anaemia.

e   Agranulocytosis.

35   Diuretics may act by

a   Increasing the blood supply to the kidney.

b   Enhancing tubular reabsorption of water by osmotic action.

c   Preventing tubular reabsorption of Na^+.

d   Inhibiting the action of aldosterone.
e   Inhibiting the action of carbonic anhydrase.

36   The following factors favour rapid and complete gastrointestinal uptake of a drug.

a   Low gastric pH.

b   Enhanced gastric emptying.

c   High lipid solubility of the drug.
d   Extensive first pass metabolism.

e   Rectal administration.

(Ch. 3, D)

a True This is recommended for urinary tract infections, 90% of which are caused by *E. Coli. (Ch. 5, BNF)*

b False This is commonly used to treat Gram-positive infections in penicillin-sensitive individuals.

c False This is used classically against Gram-positive cocci.

d True This is a late-generation penicillin, active against Gram-negative organisms. *(Ch. 5, BNF)*

e True This is active against both Gram-negative and Gram-positive bacteria but is used classically against *Haemophilus influenzae*.

(Ch. 3, D)

a False Suphonamides may cause Stevens-Johnson syndrome, but not nephrotic syndrome.

b False VIIIth nerve lesions are associated normally with aminoglycoside toxicity.

c True Modern sulphonamides are less likely to cause this.

d True Particularly if used in the presence of glucose-6-phosphate dehydrogenase deficiency, which is a contraindication.

e True

(Ch. 14, A & S; Ch. 5, D)

a False Although dopamine increases urine output as a result of renal artery dilatation, it is not usually classified as a diuretic.

b False Osmotic diuretics (e.g. mannitol) restrict reabsorption of water from the tubules because of high osmolality.

c True Diuretics of high potency (e.g. frusemide) inhibit sodium reabsorption in the proximal tubule and loop of Henle. Low potency diuretics (e.g. acetazolamide) act mainly on the distal tubule.

d True Spironolactone is an aldosterone antagonist.

e True Thiazide diuretics act here, but their main action is on the distal tubule.

(Ch. 8, A & S)

a False Little gastric absorption occurs because the surface area is low in comparison with the small intestine. No significant benefit is gained from alterations in gastric pH.

b True This is the most important factor as most absorption takes place in the small intestine.

c True This is important for diffusion to take place across the mucosa.

d False Extensive first pass metabolism reduces the bioavailability of the drug.

e True Absorption takes place via both systemic and portal venous systems.

37   **Frusemide**

   a   May cause deafness.

   b   Has a duration of action of 10 hours when given orally.
   c   May lead to decreased plasma potassium concentration.
   d   Produces a diuresis which is proportional to GFR.

   e   Raises plasma uric acid concentrations.

38   **The following are true**

   a   Tetracyclines cause discolouration and hypoplasia of growing teeth.
   b   Chloramphenicol is a bacteriostatic antibiotic.

   c   Aminoglycosides may produce neuromuscular block.

   d   Probenecid prevents tubular secretion of cephalosporins and promotes higher blood concentrations of the antibacterial agent.
   e   A dose of 30 g of benzylpenicillin can be given with impunity to an adult.

39   **Gentamicin**

   a   Is absorbed well from gastric mucosa.

   b   Is an aminoglycoside

   c   Causes VIIIth nerve injury.

   d   May cause neuromuscular blockade.

   e   May cause renal damage.

(Ch. 5, D)

a True Large doses of frusemide given rapidly may cause transient deafness. *(Ch. 2, BNF)*
b False The duration of action of oral frusemide is normally 4–6 hours.
c True Frusemide enhances potassium excretion in the kidney.
d False The diuresis produced by frusemide is inversely related to GFR. Frusemide is effective at low glomerular filtration rates. *(Ch. 14, A & S)*
e True It shares this property with bumetanide, ethacrynic acid and the thiazide diuretics

---

(Ch. 3, D; Ch. 5 BNF)

a True They are contraindicated where new bone is being laid down, such as in children.
b True This is described as bacteriostatic in low doses but bactericidal in larger doses.
c True These act as antagonists at the neuromuscular junction in a fashion similar to curare. Potentiation of curare-like drugs has been reported only with large doses of neomycin given intraperitoneally. *(Ch. 12, A & S)*
d True This is excreted preferentially rather than beta-lactam antibiotics. This prolongs the effect of the antibiotics. *(Ch. 8, A & S)*
e False The recommended maximum daily dose is 24 g in divided doses.

(Ch. 3, D)

a False In a common with other aminoglycosides, it is not absorbed and must be given parenterally.
b True Other aminoglycosides include streptomycin, kanamycin, tobramycin, netilmicin, amikacin and neomycin.
c True Ototoxicity and nephrotoxicity are side effects shared by all of these agents.
d True This is a theoretical interaction which seems to be unimportant clinically. *(Appx. 1, BNF)*.
e True The combination of frusemide and aminoglycoside antibiotics is particularly nephrotoxic.

40 **There is a decreased likelihood of placental transfer of a drug if it**
  a   Is lipid insoluble.
  b   Has a molecular weight greater than 600.

  c   Is metabolised slowly.

  d   Is highly ionised.
  e   Is administered in small doses.

---

41 **Methohexitone**
  a   Has a pH less than 8 in a 1% solution.
  b   Is a methylated barbiturate.

  c   Has a longer duration of action than that of thiopentone.
  d   Does not cause pain on i.v. injection.
  e   Is associated with fewer excitatory phenomena than thiopentone.

---

42 **Histamine causes**
  a   An increase in arterial pressure.
  b   Increased gastrointestinal motility.
  c   Bronchoconstriction.
  d   Pupillary dilation.
  e   Stimulation of the central nervous system.

---

43 **Sulphonylureas**
  a   Displace insulin from beta-cells in the pancreas.
  b   Can be used in the treatment of ketosis.
  c   Are highly protein bound.
  d   Include metoclopramide amongst the group.

  e   May lead to acidosis.

---

44 **The following pairs comprise an agonist and a competitive antagonist.**
  a   Morphine and naloxone.
  b   Histamine and promethazine.

  c   Phenobarbitone and doxapram.

  d   Acetylcholine and gallamine.
  e   Hexamethonium and methoxamine.

(Ch. 6, A & S)

a **True** Drugs must be soluble in lipid membranes to cross the placenta.
b **True** Small molecular weight compounds cross the placental barrier more readily.
c **False** A slowly metabolised drug has higher blood concentrations and a greater diffusion gradient for a longer period than one which is metabolised rapidly.
d **True** Highly ionised drugs are less lipid soluble.
e **False** Placental transfer depends more upon plasma concentration and pKa of the drug than dose.

(Ch. 10, A & S)

a **False** 1% methohexitone has a pH of approximately 11.
b **True** The methyl group is substituted in the 1 position of the barbiturate ring.
c **False**
d **False** Pain on injection occurs commonly.
e **False** Excitatory phenomena occur more commonly with methohexitone.

(Ch. 5, A & S)

a **False** It produces peripheral vasodilatation and systemic hypotension.
b **True** Because of smooth muscle contraction.
c **True** Anatomical dead-space is decreased. (Ch. 2, A & S)
d **False** Histamine has no effect upon pupillary diameter.
e **False** Although histamine receptors do exist in the central nervous system.

(Ch. 12, D)

a **True**
b **False** They are inappropriate for the treatment of ketosis or keto-acidosis
c **True** This accounts for their long half-life.
d **False** Chlorpropamide is an example of the sulphonylureas – metoclopramide is a dopamine antagonist.
e **False** Lactic acidosis may occur with the biguanides.

(Ch. 8, A & S)

a **True**
b **True** Promethazine is a phenothiazine and possesses potent H receptor blocking actions. (Ch. 11, A & S)
c **False** Doxapram is an analeptic agent and causes central nervous system stimulation. It may reverse effects of phenobarbitone, but in a non-competitive manner. (Ch. 11, A & S)
d **True** (Ch. 12, A & S)
e **False** Methoxamine is a direct acting alpha-agonist; hexamethonium is a ganglion-blocking drug.

45 **The following drugs have adverse effects on bone marrow**

   a Nitrous oxide in prolonged administration.

   b Phenylbutazone.
   c Phenytoin.

   d Phenobarbitone.
   e Paracetamol.

46 **The initial actions of intravenous mannitol include**

   a Increased blood viscosity.
   b Increased haematocrit.

   c Expansion of the blood volume.
   d Haemolysis.

   e Reduction of extracellular volume.

47 **The following antibiotics may be administered orally**

   a Cefotaxime.

   b Kanamycin.
   c Vancomycin.

   d Ticarcillin.

   e Flucloxacillin.

48 **Jaundice has been associated with administration of the following**

   a Diethyl ether.
   b Trichloroethylene.

   c Halothane.

   d Enflurane.

   e Methoxyflurane.

a True   Caused by inhibition of methionine synthetase activity.
(Ch. 9, A & S))
b True   This may cause agranulocytosis and aplastic anaemia. *(Ch. 10, BNF)*
c True   This has been reported, but megaloblastic anaemia because of folate
deficiency is the commonest problem. *(Ch. 4, BNF)*
d False
e False   Although methionine depletion has been reported, there was no
depression of bone marrow function. *(Ch. 17, D)*

(Ch. 38, A & S)

a False   Dilution of intravascular fluid causes a decrease in blood viscosity.
b False   Initially, water is drawn from the intracellular to the extracellular
space, thereby raising plasma volume and reducing haematocrit.
c True   See **b**.
d False   The hyperosmolarity of mannitol results in red cell shrinkage, not
haemolysis.
e True   See **b**.

(Ch. 3, D; Ch. 5, BNF)

a False   This is a third-generation cephalosporin which is administered only
by intramuscular or intravenous injection.
b False   This is an aminogylcoside which is inactive after oral administration.
c True   Although this is available orally, parenteral administration is the
method of choice. It is employed frequently for prophylaxis of
bacterial endocarditis preoperatively *(Appx. IV, A & S)*
d False   This is the successor to carbenicillin. It is used parenterally against
pseudomonas infections.
e True   This is the oral antistaphylococcal drug of choice.

(Ch. 9, A & S)

a True
b True   Jaundice has not been reported as a result specifically of anaesthesia
with trichloroethylene. This agent has been withdrawn from clinical
anaesthetic practice, but reports of liver damage have been
associated with its use in industry as a degreasing agent.
c True   Jaundice may be associated with the use of halothane (especially
after repeated exposure within a short space of time).
d True   Although rarer than with halothane, liver failure and jaundice have
been reported following enflurane administration.
e True   Some cases of massive hepatic necrosis have been reported,
although there is no evidence of a specific hepatotoxic effect.
Methoxyflurane has been withdrawn from the UK market.

49 **The following drugs may act on the chemoreceptor trigger zone (CTZ)**

    a Digoxin.

    b Droperidol.

    c Morphine.

    d Metoclopramide.

    e Hyoscine.

50 **The following agents decrease arterial pressure by a central action**

    a Hexamethonium.
    b Propranolol.
    c Amyl nitrate.

    d Clonidine.
    e Tubocurarine.

51 **Methaemoglobinaemia may follow administration of**

    a Sodium citrate.
    b Methylene blue.
    c Procaine.
    d Prilocaine.

    e Cinchocaine.

52 **Heparin**

    a Is a synthetic acid.
    b Is found in mast cells.

    c Is released during anaphylactic shock.
    d Is an antiplasmin.

    e May lead to osteoporosis with prolonged treatment.

a False This commonly causes loss of appetite, nausea and vomiting, but not from an effect upon the CTZ.

b True This is a specific dopamine antagonist which acts at the CTZ and is a powerful anti-emetic. *(Ch. 11, A & S)*

c True This depresses the CNS generally but stimulates the CTZ and the Edinger-Westphal nucleus (miosis). *(Ch. 1, A & S)*

d True This has peripheral actions which enhance gastric emptying, and a specific dopamine antagonistic effect on the CTZ. *(Ch. 14, A & S)*

e False This is a central nervous system depressant and an anticholinergic; it has anti-emetic actions but no direct effect upon the CTZ.

(Ch. 37.A & S)

a False This is a ganglion blocker.

b False This agent possesses negative inotropic properties.

c False This acts directly on precapillary sphincters and capacitance vessels. *(Ch. 14, A & S)*

d True *(Ch. 2, BNF)*

e False This reduces arterial pressure by a combination of ganglion blockade and histamine release.

---

a False

b False This is the agent of choice for treatment of methaemoglobinaemia.

c False

d True This produces o-toluidine leading to methaemoglobinaemia, but only if doses considerably in excess of 600 mg are administered. *(Ch. 15, A & S)*

e False

(Ch. 13, D)

a False Heparin is a complex polysaccharide.

b True It is one of the agents released in anaphylactic shock from the degranulation of the mast cell in response to stimulation of reaginic antibodies. *(Ch. 2, D)*

c True See **b**.

d False Heparin is not an antiplasmin. It accelerates the action of antithrombin III; measurement of antithrombin III activity is a method of monitoring heparin therapy.

e True Heparin is seldom used for more than two weeks because of this complication.

53 **The following are positive inotropes**

a Isoprenaline.

b Aminophylline.

c Fenfluramine.
d Methoxamine.
e Enalapril.

54 **Hypoglycaemia occurs after administration of**

a Glucagon.

b Tolbutamide.
c Diazoxide.
d Hydrocortisone.

e Propranolol.

55 **The following are beta-blockers**

a Diltiazem.
b Oxprenolol.

c Chlorpromazine.
d Salbutamol.
e Metoprolol.

56 **Bronchodilation is produced by**

a Atropine.

b Methohexitone.
c Ephedrine.

d Tubocurarine.

e Oxprenolol.

(Ch. 13, A & S)

a **True** This is a beta-agonist which stimulates both the cardiac beta$_1$- and bronchial beta$_2$-receptors.

b **True** This stimulates cAMP; it is a positive chronotrope and inotrope with a dominant action on beta$_2$-receptors.

c **False** Fenfluramine is an appetite suppressant.

d **False** Methoxamine is an alpha$_1$-adrenoceptor agonist.

e **False** Enalapril is an angiotensin-converting-enzyme inhibitor.

(Ch. 12, D)

a **False** This is produced by the alpha cells of the pancreas, and increases blood glucose concentration.

b **True** This is a suphonylurea oral hypoglycaemic agent.

c **False** This is a vasodilator which causes hyperglycaemia. *(Ch. 2, BNF)*

d **False** This enhances gluconeogenesis and glycogenolysis and therefore causes hyperglycaemia.

e **True** This may block the response to hyperglycaemia; although propranolol is not contraindicated absolutely in diabetics, a cardioselective beta-blocker is preferable. *(Ch. 2, BNF)*

(Ch. 13, A & S)

a **False** This is a calcium channel blocker.

b **True** This is a beta-blocking agent with partial agonist activity and a membrane stabilising effect.

c **False** This has alpha-adrenergic blocking actions but no beta-effects.

d **False** This is a beta$_2$-agonist.

e **True** This is cardioselective and has a membrane stabilising effect.

(Ch. 13, A & S)

a **True** Bronchoconstriction is a muscarinic effect of acetylcholine and is antagonised by atropine.

b **False**

c **True** Ephedrine is a directly and indirectly acting sympathomimetic agent.

d **False** This causes release of histamine and is contraindicated in asthmatics. *(Ch. 12, A & S)*

e **False** Oxprenolol is a beta-adrenergic blocking drug which is not cardioselective; consequently, it may cause bronchoconstriction.

57 **Drugs whose actions are reduced in the presence of hepatic enzyme induction include**

a Fentanyl.
b Phenobarbitone.

c Diazepam.
d Halothane.

e Warfarin.

58 **Thrombophlebitis may follow i.v. administration of**

a Methohexitone.
b Propofol.

c Thiopentone.

d Diazepam.

e Atracurium.

59 **Duration of action of the barbiturates is decreased by**

a Substitution of sulphur for oxygen in the 2 position.

b Methylation in the 1 or 3 position.

c Formation of sodium salts.

d Branching of carbon chains in the 5 position.

e Desaturation of carbon chain.

60 **The clearance of a drug**

a Is equal to the liver blood flow.

b Is the same for all drugs with first order kinetics.
c May be calculated from the area under the plasma concentration-time curve (AUC).
d Is equal to the infusion rate at steady state.
e Has the units of reciprocal time.

(Ch. 8, A & S)

a False The action of fentanyl is terminated by redistribution.
b True Phenobarbitone is long acting, and liver metabolism is responsible for terminating its action. Phenobarbitone causes enzyme induction.
c False Diazepam has a pharmacologically active metabolite.
d False Halothane metabolites may be responsible for toxicity. Metabolites are more likely in the presence of enzyme induction.
e True The dose may require frequent adjustment in the presence of an enzyme-inducing drug.

(Ch. 10, A & S)

a True
b False This is remarkably devoid of venous thrombotic sequelae or perivascular reactions, but pain on injection is common.
c True Although uncommon, this does occur. In addition, extravascular injection may result in tissue necrosis.
d True Venous sequelae are very common after i. v. diazepam unless the lipid formulation (Diazemuls) is used.
e False No association has been demonstrated between venous thrombosis and use of atracurium.

(Ch. 10, A & S)

a True This enhances lipid solubility and confers rapidity of onset with short duration of action.
b True Methylation particularly in the 1 position produces a rapidly acting drug with a short duration of action, but convulsive activity is more likely.
c False All the intravenous barbiturates are formulated as sodium salts in order to improve solubility.
d True Alterations in the 5 position affect potency. Increase in potency and decrease in duration of action are produced by increasing the length of the side chains or by branching of side chains.
e True Double bonds in the side chains are metabolised more easily.

(Ch. 8, A & S)

a False Clearance is the sum of all clearances including liver, renal, pulmonary, etc.
b False
c True In a two-compartment model, clearance = dose/AUC.

d False At steady state, clearance = infusion rate/plasma concentration.
e False The units are volume of plasma/time.

61   The following are available in a fat emulsion

a   Propofol.

b   Alphaxolone.

c   Ketamine.
d   Diazepam.
e   Midazolam.

62   Hartmann's solution contains

a   Sodium 112 mmol/litre.
b   Chloride 131 mmol/litre.
c   Bicarbonate 29 mmol/litre.

d   Calcium 2.4 mmol/litre.

e   Potassium 1.5 mmol/litre.

63   Oxprenolol

a   May cause increased airway resistance.

b   Decreases peripheral blood flow.
c   May cause hypoglycaemia.

d   May be used to treat symptoms of thyrotoxicosis.

e   Has a bioavailability of less than 50%.

64   Lignocaine

a   May exhibit tachyphylaxis if used as an epidural infusion.
b   Does not cross the placenta.
c   Is lipid soluble as a base but water soluble as the hydrochloride.

d   Does not depress smooth muscle.
e   Is anticonvulsant.

(Ch. 10, A & S)

a True This is prepared as an emulsion in 10% Intralipid in a concentration of 10 mg/ml.
b False This is the active constituent of Althesin (now withdrawn) and was dissolved in Cremophor-EL.
c False This is available in aqueous acidic solution.
d True Diazemuls is diazepam 5 mg/ml in Intralipid.
e False This is a water-soluble benzodiazepine. *(Ch. 11, A & S)*

(Appx. VI, A & S)

a False It contains 131 mmol/litre of sodium.
b False It contains 112 mmol/litre of chloride.
c False It contains 29 mmol/litre of lactate, which is converted to bicarbonate by the liver. Bicarbonate is precipitated in the presence of calcium.
d True This approximates to the normal plasma concentration of calcium.
e False It contains 5 mmol/litre of potassium.

(Ch. 13, A & S; Ch. 7, D)

a True $Beta_2$-blockade causes bronchiolar constriction and an increase in airway resistance.
b True This results from unopposed alpha-receptor stimulation.
c False It may aggravate diabetes mellitus by provoking hyperglycaemia. In addition, the response to hypoglycaemia may be impaired.
d True Beta-blockers are effective in the treatment of the symptoms of thyrotoxicosis but do not influence thyrotoxicosis.
e True There is significant first pass metabolism but this is offset by the production of active metabolites.

(Ch. 15, A & S)

a True All local anaesthetics have a tendency to exhibit tachyphylaxis.
b False All local anaesthetic agents cross the placenta.
c True It is presented as the hydrochloride because the basic form is lipid soluble.
d True It does not have any direct vasoconstrictor or vasodilator action.
e True Although toxic manifestations include convulsions, these are caused by cortical depression; inherently, it is a central nervous system depressant.

65 Atropine
a Exhibits more cardiac effects than hyoscine.
b Is more sedative than hyoscine.
c Is a more effective antisialagogue than glycopyrrolate.

d Causes hyperpyrexia in overdosage.

e Reduces physiological dead space.

66 Dopamine antagonists
a Cause extrapyramidal side-effects.

b May be used as anti-emetics.

c May increase gastric emptying.

d Cause tachycardia.

e May cause peripheral vasoconstriction.

67 Atracurium
a Is metabolised solely by Hoffman degradation.

b Is metabolised to laudanosine.

c Causes neuromuscular block which is prolonged by hypothermia.

d Causes neuromuscular block which is prolonged by low pH.
e Does not release histamine.

68 Alfentanil
a Is cardiodepressant.
b Is more potent than fentanyl.

c Is more lipid soluble than fentanyl.
d Has a shorter elimination half-life than fentanyl.

e Is antagonised by naloxone.

a True
b False Hyoscine is more sedative, especially in the elderly subject.
c False Glycopyrronium bromide is a quaternary amine with antisialagogue properties which are more pronounced than those of atropine.
d True The use of atropine is contraindicated in the presence of pyrexia, especially in children.
e False Physiological dead space is increased by 20%.

a True Agents such as the phenothiazines and butyrophenones are notable for extrapyramidal side-effects.
b True Dopamine antagonists have a powerful action on the CTZ (chemoreceptor trigger zone) which is physiologically outwith the blood/brain barrier.
c True Domperidone and metoclopramide are dopamine antagonists which increase the rate of gastric emptying and the tone of the lower oesophageal sphincter.
d False Dopamine antagonists do not cause tachycardia per se. However, some dopamine antagonists (e.g. chlorpromazine) also effect alpha-receptor blockade and this may lead to a tachycardia secondary to vasodilatation.
e False Some dopamine antagonists may cause vasodilatation by alpha-adrenergic blocking actions.

a False It is metabolised by ester hydrolysis in addition to Hoffman degradation.
b True This is one of the breakdown products of atracurium. However, not all of an administered dose is converted to this compound.
c True Breakdown of atracurium is slower in the presence of hypothermia and accelerated by hyperthermia.
d True Breakdown is decreased in an acid environment.
e False Histamine release is not uncommon in association with administration of atracurium.

a False Alfentanil is not cardiodepressant per se.
b False It has a much more rapid onset than other opioids but is less potent (ratio = 4:1) than fentanyl.
c True
d True The elimination half-life of fentanyl is 4 h, whereas that of alfentanil is 1.5 h. However, clearance of fentanyl is three times that of alfentanil.
e True Naloxone antagonises the actions of all u-receptor agonists.

69   Diamorphine

    a Is more potent than morphine.

    b Cannot be used in terminal care because of tolerance.

    c Causes more euphoria than morphine.

    d Is a potent cough suppressant.

    e Is a constituent of opium.

70   Vecuronium

    a Causes bradycardia.

    b Has a steroid structure.

    c Is contraindicated in the presence of renal failure.

    d Does not release histamine.

    e Contains two quaternary nitrogen groups.

71   Human albumin solution (HAS)

    a Is stored at room temperature.

    b Is prepared from pooled blood and may transmit hepatitis B.

    c Contains not less than 40g/ litre of protein.

    d Is used to treat disseminated intravascular coagulation (DIC).

    e Contains approximately 150 mmol/litre of sodium.

72   Methohexitone

    a Is an anticonvulsant.

    b Is less potent than thiopentone.

    c Is associated with hiccups.

    d Contains branched side chains in the molecule.

    e Is made up in a 10% solution.

(Ch. 11, A & S)

a **True** Diamorphine is 2–3 times more potent than morphine.
b **False** Tolerance does occur, but this is not usually a consideration in terminal care as the dose is increased if necessary.
c **True**
d **True** All opioids are effective antitussive agents.
e **False** Diamorphine is a condensation product of acetic acid and morphine. It is not a constituent of opium.

(Ch. 12, A & S)

a **False** Vecuronium has no actions on the heart. Bradycardia may occur intraoperatively as a result of surgical manipulation.
b **True** However, it possesses no hormonal activity.
c **False** It is metabolised by the liver to inactive metabolites.
d **True**
e **False** However, the second tertiary nitrogen is capable of attracting a hydrogen ion in vivo.

(Ch. 7, Appx. VI, A & S)

a **True** It has a 3-year shelf life at room temperature.
b **False** It is heat treated and this inactivates the hepatitis B virus.
c **True** It contains approximately 45 g/litre of protein.
d **False** It is low in coagulation factors.
e **True**

(Ch. 10, A & S)

a **True** Methohexitone is a cerebral depressant. There is an increased incidence of spontaneous muscle movement, but frank convulsions are not seen with methohexitone.
b **False** Methohexitone is normally used in a dose of 1–1.5 mg/kg. The induction dose of thiopentone is 4–6 mg/kg.
c **True** Hiccups are one of the manifestations of spontaneous muscle activity seen with methohexitone.
d **True** The chemical name is 1-methyl, 5-allyl, 5-(1-methyl, 2-pentyl) barbiturate.
e **False** Metholhexitone is presented as powder and is made up as a 1% solution.

73 **The action of suxamethonium is prolonged by**

a Lignocaine.
b Propofol.
c Ecothiopate.

d Neostigmine.
e Nitrogen mustard gas.

---

74 **Tachyphylaxis is exhibited clinically by**

a Ephedrine.

b Thiopentone.

c Neostigmine.
d Lignocaine.

e Suxamethonium.

---

75 **Beta-blocking drugs**

a Become less beta-selective with increasing dose.

b Are contraindicated in heart failure.

c Are classified as Vaughan-Williams group III.

d Are indicated in the treatment of supraventricular tachycardia (SVT).
e May cause peripheral vasoconstriction.

---

76 **Digitalis is employed commonly for treatment of**

a Atrial flutter.
b Idioventricular rhythm.
c Ventricular tachycardia.
d Cardiac tamponade.
e 2:1 atrioventricular block.

(Ch. 12, A & S)

a **False**
b **False**
c **True** This is an anticholinesterase used as eye drops but with systemic activity.
d **True** This is an anticholinesterase.
e **False** This is a direct cytotoxic agent. Some of the chemical warfare compounds are organophosphorus anticholinesterases, the actions of which are not easily reversible. *(Ch. 6, D)*

(Ch. 8, A & S)

a **True** This has both direct and indirect adrenoceptor agonist properties. It is thought that depletion of catecholamines at the nerve endings is responsible for tachyphylaxis.
b **False** Although acute tolerance is a feature, cumulation of drug masks this effect when multiple doses are administered.
c **False**
d **True** This is thought to be caused by saturation of intraneural buffering capacity resulting in a reduced proportion of free base.
(Ch. 15, A & S)
e **True** *(Ch. 12, A & S)*

(Ch. 13, A & S; Ch. 7, D)

a **True** As with all agents acting on the sympathetic nervous system, beta-blocking drugs become less specific with increasing dosage.
b **True** Beta-blocking drugs worsen heart failure by decreasing myocardial contractility.
c **False** Beta-blocking drugs comprise group II of the Vaughan Williams classification of anti-arrhythmic drugs. Group III comprise those drugs delaying repolarisation, such as amiodarone.
d **True** They are very effective in the treatment of SVT. *(Ch. 2, BNF)*

e **True** However, the mechanism causing this is unclear. *(Ch. 2, BNF)*

(Ch. 7, D)

a **True** It is used to control the ventricular rate.
b **False** A pacemaker is the most appropriate therapy for this condition.
c **False** It is indicated for supraventricular arrhythmias.
d **False**
e **False** It depresses atrioventricular conduction and therefore increases the block.

77 **Cocaine**

a Causes pupillary constriction.
b Is a drug of dependence.

c Is a synthetic drug.
d Is employed as a 10% solution.

e is an ester.

78 **Bupivacaine** _Marcaine_

a Has a duration of action longer than that of lignocaine.
b Is contraindicated in intravenous regional anaesthesia (IVRA).

c Is metabolised mainly by the liver.
d Is more cardiotoxic than lignocaine.

e Is available in solutions containing 1:100 000 adrenaline.

79 **The following drugs undergo significant metabolism in the liver**

a Pethidine.
b Lignocaine.

c Halothane.

d Noradrenaline.

e Chlorpromazine. — _Tardive_

80 **The following produce marked systemic analgesia**

a Droperidol. —
b Perphenazine.
c Promethazine.
d Nalbuphine.
e Fentanyl.

93

(Ch. 15, A & S)

a **False**   It has sympathomimetic properties and causes pupillary dilation.
b **True**   It is a controlled drug governed by Schedule 2 of the Misuse of
              Drugs Regulations (BNF).
c **False**   It is the alkaloid of the coca plant.
d **False**   Cocaine is available as a 1–4% solution. It was available as a 10%
              paste.
e **True**   It is a benzoic acid ester.

(Ch. 15, A & S)

a **True**   It has a duration of action 2–4 times greater than that of lignocaine.
b **True**   It is contraindicated in IVRA because of marked cardiovascular
              depression which can occur after bolus intravenous injections.
c **True**   Bupivacaine is an amide and is metabolised mainly by the liver.
d **True**   The toxic dose is 2 mg/ kg and bupivacaine produces cardiotoxicity
              before CNS depression.
e **False**   Preparations of bupivacaine are available with 1:200 000 or
              1:400 000 adrenaline (50 µg/ml and 25 µg/ml respectively).

(Ch. 8, A & S)

a **True**   It is demethylated in the liver.
b **True**   This is an amide and undergoes metabolism in the liver.
              (Ch. 15, A & S)
c **True**   Approx. 20% of an inhaled dose of halothane undergoes metabolism
              in the liver by various mechanisms, including oxidation and reduction.
              (Ch. 9, A & S)
d **False**   It is metabolised mainly at the nerve terminals by catechol-o-methyl
              transferase. Only a small proportion of noradrenaline secreted by
              nerve terminals enters the circulation and is metabolised by the
              liver.*(Ch. 13, A & S)*
e **True**   It undergoes a phase 1 reaction in the liver resulting in
              pharmacologically active metabolites. It may cause jaundice of a
              cholestatic type.

(Ch. 11, A & S)

a **False**   This is a butyrophenone.
b **False**   This is a phenothiazine.
c **False**   This is a phenothiazine.
d **True**   This is a µ-antagonist but a Kappa-agonist.
e **True**   This is a synthetic opioid analgesic derived from pethidine.

81   Pentazocine

a   Is equipotent with morphine in its analgesic effects.
b   Is antagonised by naloxone.
c   Is an opioid receptor antagonist.
d   Causes hallucinations.
e   Is a drug of dependence.

82   The following drugs are associated with spontaneous muscle movements

a   Methohexitone.

b   Diazepam.
c   Haloperidol.

d   Perphenazine.
e   Suxamethonium.

83   Morphine

a   Increases intrabiliary pressure.
b   Reduces urine output.
c   Releases histamine.
d   Is associated with neutropenia in prolonged use.

e   Causes increased baroreceptor traffic.

84   The action of non-depolarising neuromuscular blocking drugs is influenced by

a   Atypical cholinesterase.
b   Gentamicin.

c   Plasma proteins.

d   Hyponatraemia.
e   Hypothermia.

a False The usual dose of pentazocine is 30 mg (c.f. morphine 10 mg).
b True
c True It is a μ antagonist but a Kappa-agonist.
d True Hallucinations are a well-recognised feature of its use.
e True It is a controlled drug (Class B).

a True Tonic and clonic movements may occur on induction, but are reduced by opioid premedication.
b False This decreases muscle tone.
c True This is a dopamine antagonist and causes extrapyramidal side-effects.
d True This is a phenothiazine.
e True This results from fasciculations which are characteristic of depolarising block.

a True
b True It stimulates release of antidiuretic hormone.
c True It acts directly on mast cells to release histamine.
d False This occurs with N_2O, not morphine. However, morphine reduces reticuloendothelial system activity and phagocytosis by white blood cells.
e False It may cause hypotension as a result of vasodilatation secondary to central depression. Decreased baroreceptor activity ensues.

a False Atypical cholinesterase affects metabolism of suxamethonium.
b True This effect was described first with intraperitoneal neomycin, another aminoglycoside.
c True Non-depolarising neuromuscular blockers are bound to plasma proteins and alterations in the concentrations of free drugs affect bioavailability.
d False Hyponatraemia has no influence.
e True Hypothermia usually prolongs the action of non-depolarising neuromuscular blockers.

85   **Thiazide diuretics may produce**

   a   Hyponatraemia.
   b   Hypokalaemic alkalosis.
   c   Hyperuricaemia.
   d   Hyperchloraemia.
   e   Weight loss.

86   **The following drugs are calcium channel blockers**

   a   Verapamil.

   b   Captopril.
   c   Propranolol.
   d   Nifedipine.
   e   Hydralazine.

87   **The following impurities may occur in nitrous oxide**

   a   Nitrogen.
   b   Nitric oxide.

   c   Nitroglycerine.

   d   Nitrogen dioxide.
   e   Metal oxides.

88   **The following drugs undergo significant biotransformation**

   a   Methoxyflurane.

   b   Halothane.

   c   Atracurium.
   d   Isoflurane.
   e   Gallamine.

(Ch. 5, D; Ch. 14, A & S)

a False Water and sodium are excreted together.
b True   Potassium loss occurs with secondary metabolic alkalosis.
c True   This is caused by interference with uric acid excretion.
d False Hypochloraemia is more common.
e True   Caused by water loss.

(Ch. 14, A & S)

a True   This was the first commercially available calcium channel blocking drug.
b False This is an angiotensin-converting-enzyme inhibitor.
c False This is a beta-adrenoceptor blocker.
d True
e False This is a direct-acting vasodilator.

(Ch. 9, A & S)

a True   Nitrogen is present in the manufacture of nitrous oxide.
b True   Nitric oxide occurs as an impurity during manufacture and is removed by 'scrubbing' with water, with which it forms nitrous acid.
c False Nitroglycerine is formed by heating glycerin with concentrated nitric acid. It is not a by-product of manufacture of nitrous oxide.
d True   This is removed by 'scrubbing' with water to form nitric acid.
e False Metal oxides are not produced from the decomposition of ammonium nitrate (NH_4NO_3).

(Ch. 9, Ch. 12, A & S)

a True   50–70% of absorbed methoxyflurane is metabolised to oxalic acid, fluoride, carbon dioxide, dichloroacetic acid and methoxyfluoroacetic acid. The first two of these metabolites have been held responsible for high output renal failure.
b True   More than 20% of halothane is metabolised normally by oxidative pathways.
c True   It undergoes spontaneous degradation at normal blood pH.
d False Less than 1% of isoflurane undergoes metabolism.
e False It is excreted almost entirely unchanged in the kidney. Its use in renal failure is contraindicated.

89   The actions of benzodiazepines

a   Result from inhibition of GABA receptors.

b   Include profound retrograde amnesia.
c   Relieve acute anxiety.
d   May result in respiratory depression.
e   Mostly result from active metabolites.

90   The pupil is dilated by instillation of the following drugs into the conjunctival sac.

a   Ephedrine.
b   Timolol.

c   Homatropine.
d   Cocaine.
e   Chloramphenicol.

91   Lithium

a   Inhibits release of noradrenaline.
b   Potentiates neuromuscular block.

c   Is excreted by the renal tubules.
d   Has a narrow therapeutic ratio.
e   Is more toxic in the presence of hypernatraemia.

92   Flumazenil

a   Antagonises the actions of lorazepam.
b   May be administered orally.
c   Does not reverse the amnesic actions of benzodiazepines.
d   Undergoes rapid metabolism in the liver.

e   Prevents the benzodiazepine withdrawal syndrome.

93   Dantrolene

a   Stimulates respiration.
b   Is a muscle relaxant.

c   Is the drug of choice for the treatment of malignant hyperthermia.
d   Is a good analgesic.
e   Antagonises benzodiazepines.

(Ch. 11, A & S)

a False The actions of the inhibitory transmitter, GABA are facilitated by benzodiazepines.
b False Anterograde amnesia only occurs.
c True This action renders the group useful for premedication.
d True Particularly on i.v. administration.
e False Diazepam has an active metabolite but other members of the group do not.

(Ch. 11, BNF)

a True Ephedrine has sympathomimetic actions.
b False Timolol is a beta-blocker used in the treatment of glaucoma; it causes pupillary constriction.
c True Homatropine has a shorter duration of action than atropine.
d True It possesses sympathomimetic actions.
e False

(Ch. 30, A & S; Ch. 4, BNF)

a True Lithium is used in the treatment of manic states.
b True It substitutes for sodium ions. Both depolarising and non-depolarising blockers may be potentiated.
c True
d True Plasma concentrations should be monitored.
e False Lithium toxicity is exacerbated by sodium depletion.

(Ch. 11, A & S; Ch, 15, BNF)

a True Flumazenil is a benzodiazepine antagonist.
b False It must be administered by i.v. bolus injection or i.v. infusion.
c False All central actions of benzodiazepines are antagonised.
d True Its elimination half-life is less than 1 h. Sedation and amnesia caused by long-acting benzodiazepines may return.
e False It may induce withdrawal symptoms after long-term use of benzodiazepines.

(Ch. 23, A & S)

a False It does not stimulate respiration.
b True It is a direct acting muscle relaxant rather than a neuromuscular blocker.
c True It should be used early and in appropriate dosage.
d False It has no analgesic activity.
e False The specific benzodiazepine antagonist is flumazenil.

94   Adrenaline

    a   Increases pulmonary ventilation.

    b   Is excreted as indole acetic acid.

    c   Dilates the pupil.
    d   Stimulates alpha adrenoreceptors.
    e   Causes diastolic hypotension.

95   Sulphonylureas.

    a   May cause lactic acidosis.

    b   Are useful in maturity onset diabetes.
    c   May produce reactive hypoglycaemia.

    d   Are useful in post-pancreatectomy patients.

    e   May cause nausea and vomiting.

96   Promethazine

    a   Is an antihistamine.

    b   Has anticholinergic actions.
    c   Is less sedative than chlorpromazine.
    d   Causes anterograde amnesia.
    e   May precipitate acute porphyria.

97   Properties of halothane include
    a   Chemical structure of C_2HF_3BrCl.
    b   Bronchoconstriction.
    c   MAC of 0.8.
    d   Good analgesia at subanaesthetic concentrations.
    e   Increase in CSF pressure.

(Ch. 13, A & S)

a True Tachypnoea is a frequent accompaniment of sympathetic stimulation.

b False Indole acetic acid is the metabolic product of 5-hydroxyindole acetic acid and 5-hydroxytryptamine. Adrenaline is excreted in the urine as 3-methoxy-4-hydroxy mandelic acid.

c True

d True It stimulates both alpha- and beta-receptors.

e False In general, adrenaline causes an increase in both peripheral resistance and cardiac output and results in hypertension. Diastolic pressure is affected less, and pulse pressure is increased.

(Ch. 12, D)

a False This is a complication of treatment with biguanides but not sulphonylureas.

b True Maturity onset diabetes is treated commonly with sulphonylureas.

c True Sulphonylureas may lead to hypoglycaemia occurring four or more hours after food and this may be an indication of overdose.

d False The sulphonylureas act mainly by augmenting the secretion of insulin.

e True Side-effects of sulphonylureas include gastrointestinal disturbances.

(Ch. 11, Ch. 14, A & S)

a True Its antihistaminic actions are more marked than those of other phenothiazines.

b True It causes bronchodilation and reduces secretions.

c False It has a greater sedative effect than chlorpromazine.

d False

e True Antihistamines, with the exception of chlorpromazine and cyclizine, should be avoided in porphyria.

(Ch. 9, A & S)

a False Halothane is CF_3 CHClBr. *(Appx. II, A & S)*

b False It is a useful agent for the asthmatic patient.

c True *(Appx. II, A & S)*

d False Unlike nitrous oxide.

e True In common with other volatile agents.

98   Naloxone antagonises the respiratory depression caused by

a   Enflurane.
b   Buprenorphine.

c   Pentazocine.
d   Phenazocine.
e   Barbiturates.

99   The following statements are true of local anaesthetics

a   The maximum safe dose of plain lignocaine is 3 mg/kg.

b   The maximum safe dose of plain bupivacaine is 2 mg/kg.
c   Amethocaine is hydrolysed by serum cholinesterase.
d   Bupivacaine is an ester-linked drug.
e   Etidocaine selectively blocks motor nerves.

100   The following are features of hyoscine but not atropine, in usual therapeutic doses

a   Anti-emetic actions.

b   Anti-Parkinsonian actions.
c   Sedation.

d   Tachycardia.
e   Mydriasis.

a False Enflurane has no effect at opioid receptors.
b True This is a partial agonist with very high affinity for μ-receptors. Very high doses of naloxone may be required, and non-specific ventilatory stimulants are preferred.
c True But pentazocine is an antagonist at μ-receptors.
d False *(Ch. 4, BNF)*
e False The mechanism of ventilatory depression caused by barbiturates is different from that of opioids. *(Ch. 10, A & S)*

---

a True But caution must be exercised where rapid intravascular injection is possible.
b True It is cardiotoxic.
c True It is a para-aminobenzoic acid derivative.
d False It is an amide and is metabolised in the liver.
e True This drug produces a more marked motor than sensory block.

---

a False Both atropine and hyoscine have anti-emetic actions but hyoscine is more potent and is used commonly as prophylaxis against motion sickness.
b False Both atropine and hyoscine exert anti-Parkinsonian effects.
c True Hyoscine frequently produces sedation and this is evident particularly in the elderly.
d False Hyoscine produces less tachycardia than atropine.
e False Atropine tends to cause more mydriasis than hyoscine.

3. Medicine

1   A patient had a preoperative serum urea concentration of 10 mmol/litre, and a serum creatinine concentration of 200 µmol/litre. Several days after cholecystectomy, the urea concentration is 22 mmol/litre and the creatinine is 240 µmol/litre; urine sodium content is 140 mmol/24 h and serum osmolality is 300 mosmol/kg. The following are true

a   The patient had disordered renal function preoperatively.
b   The patient is now dehydrated.

c   Intravenous fluids should be given.

d   The likely diagnosis is an acute exacerbation of chronic renal failure.
e   Measurement of creatinine clearance is indicated.

2   Endotoxic septicaemia

a   Is always produced by Gram-negative organisms.
b   Is associated usually with positive blood culture.

c   Is associated always with a low cardiac output.
d   Has a good prognosis.
e   Is relatively common after genito-urinary surgery.

3   In carbon monoxide poisoning the following are seen

a   Arrhythmias.
b   Hypotension.
c   Extensor plantar reflexes.
d   Cyanosis.
e   Cerebral oedema.

(Ch. 4, Appx. X, A & S)

a True The serum urea and creatinine concentrations were high.
b False The urinary sodium concentration and serum osmolality are within normal limits.
c False Careful clinical assessment is necessary before i.v. fluid therapy. *(Ch. 41, A & S)*
d True The serum urea concentration may increase rapidly postoperatively if chronic renal failure is present. *(Ch. 41, A & S)*
e True This would confirm the loss of renal function. *(Ch. 11, D)*

(Ch. 42, A & S)

a False Gram-positive organisms may be implicated in some cases.
b False Blood culture does not always yield positive results and antibiotic treatment should not be withheld.
c False Cardiac output may be elevated, especially in the early phase.
d False Mortality may be greater than 60%.
e False But genito-urinary surgery is a common source of infection in bacteraemic shock. *(Ch. 3, D)*

(p. 1104, D [10th ed])

a True Ectopic beats and atrial fibrillation are common.
b True Heart failure and hypotension may develop rapidly.
c True This occurs if poisoning is severe.
d False Classically, a cherry red colour is evident.
e True This contributes to eventual coma.

4   The following are associated with haemophilia

   a Haemarthrosis.
   b Mucous membrane haemorrhages.

   c Haemorrhagic rash.
   d Decreased clot retraction.
   e Positive Schilling test.

5   The following may be used in the presence of reversible airways obstruction

   a Metoprolol.
   b Practolol.
   c Pethidine.

   d Helium.
   e Propranolol.

6   Tension pneumothorax

   a Is accompanied by deviation of the trachea to the opposite side.
   b Is a risk of spinal cord surgery.
   c Is accompanied by stridor.

   d Results in a decreased arterial P_{O_2}.

   e Is treated by tracheal intubation and positive pressure ventilation.

7   The following are features of chronic constrictive pericarditis

   a Raised jugular venous pulse (JVP) which decreases during inspiration.
   b An association with chronic uraemia.
   c Atrial enlargement.

   d Reduced cardiac diameter on chest X-ray.

   e Pericardial friction rub.

(Ch. 13, D)

a True Haemarthrosis is a well-recognised complication of haemophilia.
b False Mucous membrane haemorrhages are not a common complication of haemophilia.
c False Haemorrhagic rash is associated commonly with platelet deficiency.
d False Clot retraction is normal in haemophilia.
e False The Schilling test assesses uptake of vitamin B_{12} from the gut.

(Ch. 13, A & S)

a True In normal doses, metoprolol is a cardioselective beta-blocker.
b False Practolol is no longer available in the UK.
c True Pethidine has mild anticholinergic actions, releases less histamine than morphine and is preferable for asthmatic patients.
(Ch. 11, A & S)
d True But there is no specific benefit in this situation.
e False Propranolol is a non-cardioselective beta-blocker.

(Ch. 32, A & S)

a True This results from positive pressure in the affected hemithorax.
b False There is no increased risk with spinal surgery. *(Ch. 38, A & S)*
c False Stridor is an indication of upper respiratory tract obstruction.
(Ch. 8, D)
d True Because of hypoventilation of the lung on the affected side and increased shunting. *(Ch. 2, A & S)*
e False An intercostal chest drain should be inserted expeditiously.

(Ch. 7, D)

a False The JVP is raised and decreases with opening of the tricuspid valve, but not on inspiration.
b False Acute pericarditis is more common.
c False The chambers of the heart may be compressed by the expanding effusion.
d False The heart shadow is not enlarged. Pericardial calcification may be evident on chest X-ray.
e False Friction rub is characteristic of acute pericarditis.

8 **Intravenous entrainment of air is hazardous particularly in patients with**

    a Patent ductus arteriosus (PDA).

    b Ventricular septal defect (VSD).

    c Pulmonary valve stenosis.

    d Patent foramen ovale.

    e Tricuspid incompetence.

9 **In respect of propranolol administration**

    a Left bundle branch block is a contraindication.

    b Hypokalaemia is a contraindication.

    c Digoxin therapy is a contraindication.

    d History of nocturnal dyspnoea is a contraindication.

    e Administration may cause postural hypotension.

10 **The following may cause liver damage in acute overdose**

    a Paracetamol.

    b Aspirin.

    c Paraquat.

    d Amitriptyline.

    e Halothane.

(Ch. 7, D)

a False Entrained air is unlikely to gain access to the systemic circulation, because the shunt is usually from left to right.
b True With a ventricular septal defect, right-to-left shunting occurs in the presence of systemic hypotension and/or pulmonary hypertension.
c False But an associated ventricular septal defect may be more dangerous in the presence of pulmonary valve stenosis.
d True Right-to-left shunting of blood may occur in the presence of pulmonary hypertension.
e False This occurs secondary to right ventricular dilatation.

(Ch. 13, A & S; Ch. 7, D)

a True Left bundle branch block may progress occasionally to complete heart block and idioventricular rhythm. Propranolol may produce bradycardia and exacerbate this tendency.
b False Hypokalaemia should be corrected but is not a contraindication to propranolol therapy.
c False Although there is a theoretical possibility of complete heart block with digoxin, in practice digoxin therapy is not a recognised contraindication to propranolol therapy. *(Ch. 2, BNF)*
d True Nocturnal dyspnoea indicates incipient heart failure. This is an important contraindication to propranolol therapy, which potentiates failure.
e True Postural hypotension may be associated with beta-blockade. A fully beta-blocked patient is unable to compensate with tachycardia in the presence of hypotension.

(Ch. 7, D)

a True This is a well-recognised side-effect which can be prevented by administration of adequate doses of methionine.
b False Liver damage is not associated with acute overdose of aspirin. *(Ch. Em, BNF)*
c False Paraquat in acute overdosage causes a severe fibrotic reaction in the lungs but not liver damage per se. *(Ch. Em, BNF)*
d False Tricyclic antidepressant agents produce anticholinergic effects in overdosage; liver damage is not a feature. *(Ch. Em, BNF)*
e False In *acute* overdosage halothane causes cardiovascular and cerebral depression. *(Ch. 9, A & S)*

11   A urine specific gravity of 1030 is compatible with

    a   Diabetes insipidus.

    b   Diabetes mellitus.

    c   Normal renal function.

    d   Methoxyflurane nephrotoxicity.

    e   Syndrome of inappropriate ADH secretion.

---

12   Metabolic acidosis may be caused by

    a   Implantation of the ureters into the colon.   *hyperchloraemic acidosis*

    b   Hypoventilation.

    c   Acute renal failure.

    d   Pancreatic fistulae.   *- loss of alkali*

    e   Chronic diarrhoea.

---

13   Aortic regurgitation is a common feature of

    a   Marfan's syndrome.

    b   Rheumatoid arthritis.

    c   Ankylosing spondylitis.

    d   Acromegaly.

    e   Thyrotoxicosis.

---

14   In a patient with intestinal obstruction there may be

    a   An increased risk of pulmonary aspiration.

    b   Hyponatraemia.

    c   Hypovolaemia.

    d   Hyperkalaemia.

    e   Stimulation of ADH secretion if dehydration is present.

a False A specific gravity of 1010 is expected in diabetes insipidus.
b True A specific gravity of 1030 is normal; in the absence of glycosuria, a patient with diabetes mellitus produces urine with normal specific gravity.
c True This value is within the normal range.
d False Methoxyflurane nephrotoxicity results in dilute urine and high-output renal failure.
e False Inappropriate secretion of ADH results in concentrated urine, with consequent water overload. *(Ch. 5, D)*

---

a True This may cause a hyperchloraemic acidosis. *(Ch. 9, D)*
b False This results in respiratory acidosis. *(Ch. 2, A & S)*
c True Metabolic acidosis is caused by inability to excrete hydrogen ions. *(Ch. 4, A & S, Ch. 11, D)*
d True Loss of pancreatic juices results in loss of alkali and consequent metabolic acidosis. *(Ch. 9, D)*
e True Acidosis secondary to loss of bicarbonate may occur with chronic diarrhoea. *(Ch. 5, D)*

(Ch. 7, D)

a True Marfan's syndrome is a connective tissue disorder characterised by long thin extremities, high arched palate and subluxation of the lens. Dilatation of the first part of the aorta may occur, leading to aortic regurgitation.
b False Although rheumatoid granuloma may lead to aortic regurgitation, this is extremely rare. *(Ch. 14, D)*
c True This is a well-recognised complication of ankylosing spondylitis. *(Ch. 14, D)*
d False Cardiac failure occurs in acromegaly but this is not associated usually with aortic regurgitation.
e False A systolic aortic flow murmur may be present in thyrotoxicosis. *(Ch. 12, D)*

(Ch. 32, A & S)

a True Vomiting, regurgitation and the possibility of aspiration always exist in a patient with intestinal obstruction.
b True Although hyponatraemia is possible, hypernatraemia or a normal serum sodium concentration is more usual in the presence of dehydration.
c True Loss of extracellular fluid into the bowel or by vomiting results in hypovolaemia.
d False If vomiting accompanies intestinal obstruction loss of potassium and metabolic alkalosis may lead to hypokalaemia.
e False Secretion of ADH accompanies the stress response. *(Ch. 8, D)*

15   In chronic obstructive airways disease (COAD)

a   The trachea descends on inspiration.

b   Finger clubbing is a feature.

c   Percussion of the heart border is an unreliable test of cardiomegaly.

d   The JVP may be raised.

e   The P wave on ECG may be abnormal.

16   The following are true of anaphylaxis

a   There is an increased incidence in atopic patients.

b   Hydrocortisone 200 mg is the first line treatment.

c   Previous exposure to the offending agent is unusual.

d   Adrenaline should be administered.

e   It is less common following oral than i.v. administration of the aetiological agent.

17   In sickle cell disease

a   Individuals have either African or West Indian ancestry.

b   The Sickledex test is negative for the trait.

c   Sickling occurs only at an oxygen tension < 2.9 kPa.

d   Sickling is promoted by acidosis.

e   The crisis is precipitated by metabolic alkalosis.

18   In acute intermittent porphyria the following drugs are contraindicated:

a   Methohexitone.

b   Sulphonamides.

c   Chlorpropamide.

d   Propofol.

e   Non-steroidal anti-inflammatory drugs (NSAIDs).

(Ch. 8, D)

a True Tracheal descent on inspiration may be a feature of severe forms of emphysema.
b False Finger clubbing is a feature of suppurative lung disease and not COAD.
c True Because of the increased anteroposterior diameter of the chest and increased resting lung volume.
d True JVP may be raised if right heart failure complicates chronic obstructive airways disease.
e True An abnormal P wave (P pulmonale) on the ECG occurs because of enlargement of the right atrium.

(Ch. 2, D)

a True In atopic patients there is an increased serum concentration of IgE.
b False Hydrocortisone has no effect on immediate outcome and should be regarded as second-line therapy. *(Ch. 3, BNF)*
c False Previous exposure to the antigen is common in an anaphylactic reaction.
d True Adrenaline 300–500 µg should be administered. *(Ch. 23, A & S)*
e True With oral administration of an agent there is 'filtering' by the gastrointestinal tract. *(Ch. 2, D)*

(Ch. 13, D; Ch. 7, A & S)

a False The sickle-cell gene is found also in those of Mediterranean origin or, less commonly, in those from the Indian subcontinent.
b False The Sickledex test is positive for both the trait (heterozygote) and the disease (homozygote).
c False Sickling in the homozygote occurs with oxygen tensions in the venous range (5–5.5 kPa).
d True Sickling is more likely to occur with low blood pH, high red cell 2, 3-DPG concentrations, stasis, dehydration and increased plasma osmolality.
e False Alkalosis is less likely to promote sickling of the abnormal red cells.

---

a True All barbiturates are contraindicated in acute intermittent porphyria (AIP). *(Ch. 10, A & S)*
b True The sulphonamides are contraindicated in AIP. *(Ch. 15, D)*
c True Chlorpropamide is a derivative of the sulphonamide group and is contraindicated in AIP. *(Ch. 15, D)*
d False Propofol does not precipitate an attack of AIP.
e False NSAIDs are regarded as safe in the presence of this disorder. *(Ch. 41, A & S)*

19   Reactions to blood transfusion usually include

a   Bronchospasm.

b   Laryngeal oedema.

c   Urticaria.

d   Facial oedema.

e   Myoglobinuria.

20   The following drugs are used currently to treat supraventricular tachycardia (SVT)

a   Verapamil.

b   Propranolol.

c   Lignocaine.

d   Nifedipine.

e   Neostigmine.

21   In acute severe hypovolaemia

a   Tidal volume increases.

b   Hyperventilation occurs.

c CO_2 retention occurs.

d   Ventilation/perfusion mismatch occurs.

e   The oxyhaemoglobin dissociation curve shifts to the right.

(Ch. 13, D; Ch. 7, A & S)

a False Most transfusion reactions are haemolytic in nature. Anaphylactic reactions may occur; release of histamine would lead to marked bronchospasm, although this is rare.

b False This is a rare complication.

c True Urticarial weals or hives are thought to result from reaction between IgA and anti-IgA.

d False This is very rare.

e False Haemoglobinuria occurs commonly because of haemolysis, but myoglobinuria, caused by destruction of muscle myoglobin, does not occur.

(Ch. 14, A & S; Ch. 2, BNF)

a True Verapamil, a calcium channel blocking drug, reduces the rate of spontaneous depolarisation.

b True Beta-blockade permits unopposed vagal activity on the sino-atrial node. *(Ch. 13, A & S)*

c False Lignocaine is a membrane stabilising drug and has no effect on supraventricular arrhythmias.

d False Although nifedipine is a calcium channel blocking drug, its predominant effects are peripheral and coronary vasodilatation.

e False Neostigmine has been superseded by modern therapy in this respect.

---

a True Increased vasomotor centre activity radiates to the respiratory centre. *(Ch. 7, D)*

b True Increased peripheral chemoreceptor activity leads to stimulation of the respiratory centre. *(Ch. 3, A & S)*

c False There is hyperventilation and a decrease in Pa_{CO_2}.

d True Increased ventilation accompanied by a reduction in cardiac output and pulmonary artery pressure leads to an increase in V/Q scatter. Oxygen therapy is important in the management of severe hypovolaemia.

e False Respiratory alkalosis shifts the oxyhaemoglobin dissociation curve to the left. *(Ch. 2, A & S)*

22   **ABO blood group antigens**

    a   Exhibit Mendelian inheritance.

    b   Are thought to be contained within red cells.

    c   Are absent in patients with blood group O.

    d   Are absent from leucocytes.
    e   May be removed by washing red cells.

23   **The following suggest acute massive pulmonary embolism**

    a   Accentuated mitral valve sounds.

    b   Elevated JVP.

    c   Deep Q waves and inverted T waves in lead I of the ECG.

    d   Cyanosis.

    e   Hepatojugular reflux.

24   **Insulin requirements increase**

    a   Following onset of chronic renal failure.

    b   During treatment with beta-blockers.

    c   During the third trimester of pregnancy.

    d   Following the onset of diabetic gangrene.

    e   During treatment with dopamine.

(Ch. 7, A & S)

a True The ABO blood groups described by Landsteiner exhibit Mendelian inheritance.

b False The antigenic elements of ABO blood groups are found on the surface of red cells.

c True The blood of group O patients contains antibodies to both A and B antigens.

d True The ABO system is a red cell system.

e False The washing of red cells is used to prevent HLA incompatibility from white cells.

(Ch. 7, D)

a False In acute massive pulmonary embolism, there is wide splitting of the second heart sound and a third sound may be heard over the right ventricle.

b True This invariably accompanies massive pulmonary embolism because of right ventricular failure.

c False The ECG may show signs of acute right ventricular strain with an S-wave in lead I and T-wave inversion in V_1.

d True The combination of severe V/Q mismatch and reduction in cardiac output results in cyanosis.

e False Hepatojugular reflux is a sign of longstanding right ventricular failure and liver congestion.

(Ch. 12, D)

a False Diabetic nephropathy may progress to chronic renal failure but diabetic management is unaffected.

b True Theoretically, beta-blockers may antagonise gluconeogenesis, but beta-blocker treatment may cause a reduction in glucose tolerance in diabetics and insulin requirements are increased.
(Ch. 2, BNF; Ch. 41, A & S)

c True Insulin requirements increase during pregnancy. After parturition there may be a rapid decline. *(Ch. 12, D)*

d True The onset of infection produces insulin resistance and requirements increase. *(Ch. 12, D)*

e True This causes an increase in circulating catecholamine concentrations and impairment of glucose tolerance.

25   Rheumatoid arthritis

a   May produce fixed flexion deformities of the neck.
b   May be associated with mitral valve disease.
c   May be associated with anaemia refractory to treatment.

d   Commonly involves the temporomandibular joint.

e   Is associated with discrete shadowing on the chest X-ray.

26   Gallstones are associated with the following

a   Haemolytic anaemia.

b   Raised serum concentrations of bile salts.

c   Raised serum concentrations of calcium.

d   Hypoparathyroidism.

e   Pancreatic carcinoma.

27   Propranolol is contraindicated preoperatively if the following are present

a   Left bundle branch block.

b   Orthopnoea or paroxysmal nocturnal dyspnoea.

c   Bronchial asthma.
d   Therapy with digoxin.

e   Therapy with verapamil.

28   Acute appendicitis may be mimicked by

a   Carcinoma of the caecum.
b   Herpes zoster.

c   Basal pneumonia.
d   Mesenteric adenitis.

e   Ectopic pregnancy.

(Ch. 41, A & S)

a **True** The cervical spine may be fixed, or subluxed. *(Ch. 27, A & S)*
b **False** Rheumatoid arthritis is unrelated to rheumatic heart disease.
c **True** Chronic anaemia, either hypo- or normochromic is common and this is refractory to iron therapy. In addition, non-steroidal anti-inflammatory drugs may cause gastrointestinal haemorrhage.
d **True** The arthritic process may involve the temporomandibular joint, rendering laryngoscopy and intubation difficult.
e **True** There may be pulmonary involvement with interstitial fibrosis producing V/Q abnormalities and hypoxaemia.

(Ch. 10, D)

a **True** This results from increased quantities of products of haemoglobin metabolism.
b **True** 25% of gallstones comprise pigment stones (calcium and bilirubinate).
c **False** Increased serum concentrations of calcium may cause renal stones. *(Ch. 11, D)*
d **False** Hypoparathyroidism leads to decreased serum concentrations of calcium; there is no association with gallstones *(Ch. 12, D)*
e **False** There is no association between pancreatic carcinoma and gallstones.

(Ch. 13, A & S)

a **True** Left bundle branch block can progress to complete heart block in the presence of beta-blockade.
b **True** Propranolol is a myocardial depressant and therefore contraindicated in the presence of left ventricular failure.
c **True** Propranolol is a non-cardioselective beta-blocker. *(Ch. 2, BNF)*
d **False** But care should be exercised in the presence of cardiac failure (see **b**).
e **True** The myocardial depressant actions of verapamil and beta-blockers are additive. *(Ch. 2, BNF)*

(Ch. 9, D)

a **True** Acute appendicitis in adults may cause a mass in the right iliac fossa.
b **True** Prodromal symptoms of herpes zoster in the right T12/L1 dermatomes may mimic the pain of acute appendicitis. *(Ch. 15, D)*
c **True** Right basal pneumonia may produce pain in the right flank.
d **True** Non-specific mesenteric lymphadenitis may resemble appendicitis in children and adolescents.
e **True** But not in men!

29   Features of thyrotoxicosis in a young adult include

a   Low pulse pressure.
b   Large goitre.
c   Cold intolerance.
d   Menorrhagia.

e   Atrial fibrillation.

30   The causes of an increase in serum urea concentration after haematemesis include

a   Catabolism of blood in the gut.
b   Potassium loss.
c   Metabolic acidosis.
d   Hypovolaemia.

e   Dehydration.

31   Hypokalaemia

a   Causes enlarged P waves on the ECG.
b   Occurs in hyperaldosteronism.

c   Is a feature of Cushing's syndrome.
d   Is a feature of Cushing's disease.
e   Always reflects a decrease in total body potassium content.

32   Hyperkalaemia may be treated with

a   Intravenous insulin.

b   Intravenous calcium.

c   Oral ion exchange resins.

d   Frusemide.

e   Glucocorticoids.

(Ch. 12, D)

a False Increased pulse pressure usually occurs.
b False There may be a goitre, but it is not usually large.
c False Cold intolerance is a feature of hypothyroidism.
d True Menorrhagia may be a presenting symptom in this condition; thyrotoxicosis is eight times more frequent in females than in males.
e True Thyrotoxicosis is a common non-cardiac cause of atrial fibrillation.

(Ch. 9, D)

a True Following red cell breakdown by intestinal bacteria.
b False Potassium loss does not influence serum urea concentration.
c False Serum urea concentration is not influenced by pH of blood.
d True Fluid loss from the extracellular space but not hypovolaemia per se causes an increase in serum urea concentration.
e True Dehydration from any cause may lead to increased serum urea concentration.

(Ch. 5, Ch. 12, D; Ch. 22, A & S)

a False Hypokalaemia causes decreased T wave amplitude.
b True Excretion of K^+ is enhanced by aldosterone. Primary hyperaldosteronism is termed Conn's syndrome.
c True Excess mineralocorticoid activity promotes K^+ excretion.
d True See **c**.
e False Hypokalaemia may be caused by compartmental shifts rather than loss from the body.

(Ch. 5, D; Ch. 22, A & S)

a True This enhances Na^+/K^+/ATP-ase activity and transfer of potassium from extra- to intracellular compartments.
b True This restores the Ca^{++}/K^+ ratio and stabilises membranes especially in cardiac muscle.
c True Calcium resonium 15 g, 6-hourly, is recommended, but is expensive and messy.
d False Although loop diuretics promote K^+ loss, this is not an initial treatment of choice. Hyperkalaemia may be the result of renal failure.
e False Glucocorticoids promote K^+ loss but this action is not adequate for therapy.

33   Aortic stenosis may be caused by

    a   Congenital anomalies.

    b   Aortic valve calcification.
    c   Ruptured aortic cusp.
    d   Endocarditis.

    e   Hypertrophic obstructive cardiomyopathy (HOCM).

34   The trachea may be deviated to the right in

    a   Right upper lobe fibrosis.
    b   Left simple pneumothorax.

    c   Right pleural effusion.

    d   Left lower lobar collapse.

    e   Retrosternal goitre.

35   The risk of DVT is increased by

    a   Bed rest.
    b   Anaemia.
    c   Neoplastic disease.
    d   Obesity.
    e   Extradural anaesthesia.

36   Atrial fibrillation is associated with

    a   Mitral stenosis.

    b   Ischaemic heart disease.

    c   Increased cardiac output.

    d   Multiple P waves on ECG.

    e   Thrombus formation in the left atrial appendage.

a True Aortic stenosis may result from premature calcification of a bicuspid aortic valve, or a subvalvular diaphragm.

b True This is common, especially in old age.

c False This results in aortic regurgitation.

d False This causes destruction of the valve leaflets, producing a systolic flow murmur and ultimately regurgitation.

e False The signs of HOCM are similar to those of aortic stenosis but the obstruction is subvalvular.

---

a False Fibrosis of the right upper lobe is unlikely to shift the trachea.

b False Deviation of the trachea to the right with a left pneumothorax occurs only if it is under tension.

c False Pleural effusions do not *usually* shift the trachea or mediastinum. However, if tracheal deviation is present, it would probably be to the left.

d False Left lower lobar collapse does not result in deviation of the trachea to the right.

e True The trachea may be deviated to left, right or not at all.

---

a True Bed rest causes venous stasis (part of Virchow's triad).

b False Polycythaemia increases the risk of DVT.

c True Especially pelvic neoplasms.

d True This results from immobility.

e False Extradural anaesthesia has not been shown to increase risk of deep venous thrombosis, and may reduce it. *(Ch. 26, A & S)*

---

a True Atrial dilatation, secondary to mitral stenosis, leads to atrial fibrillation.

b True Atrial fibrillation may be a sign of ischaemic heart disease in elderly patients.

c False Atrial contraction contributes approximately 20% to ventricular filling; cardiac output is reduced in atrial fibrillation.

d False Fibrillary waves characterise atrial fibrillation. P waves represent ordered depolarisation.

e True Anticoagulant therapy may be advisable.

37   Hyperkalaemia is associated with

    a   Tall peaked T waves on the ECG.

    b   U waves on the ECG.

    c   Enhanced digoxin toxicity.

    d   Pyloric stenosis.

    e   Haemolysis.

---

38   In chronic renal failure

    a   The patient is symptomless until the glomerular filtration rate is less than 15 ml/min.

    b   Anaemia is common and must be corrected before surgery.

    c   Hypertension occurs because of secondary hyperaldosteronism.

    d   Suxamethonium is contraindicated because of hyperkalaemia.

    e   Enflurane is the volatile agent of choice during anaesthesia.

---

39   Serum concentrations of Na$^+$ 127 mmol/litre, K$^+$ 6.0 mmol/litre, urea 18 mmol/litre, glucose 3 mmol/litre, NaHCO$_3$ 18 mmol/litre are compatible with

    a   Renal failure.

    b   Addison's disease.

    c   Inappropriate secretion of ADH.

    d   Liver failure.

    e   Fluid overload.

---

40   In hepatocellular insufficiency the following occur

    a   Hypokalaemia.

    b   Decreased plasma albumin concentration.

    c   Raised plasma bilirubin concentration.

    d   Decreased prothrombin time.

    e   Hyponatraemia.

(Ch. 22, A & S)

a **True** Hyperkalaemia decreases the resting membrane potential. Tall T waves are an early indication of an increased serum potassium concentration.

b **False** 'U' waves are associated with hypokalaemia.

c **False** Hyperkalaemia ameliorates digoxin toxicity.

d **False** Hypokalaemia may occur secondary to metabolic alkalosis.
(Ch. 34, A & S)

e **True** Because of release of intracellular potassium.

(Ch. 11, D)

a **True** Slow deterioration of renal function may not be accompanied by symptoms until a late stage in the disease.

b **False** Anaemia, though common, is well compensated, and preoperative transfusion should not be necessary. Prompt treatment of intraoperative blood loss should take place.

c **True** Fluid retention also contributes. Patients often require antihypertensive medication.

d **True** Further potassium release may occur, which is more hazardous in the hyperkalaemic patient.

e **False** Enflurane is metabolised with the liberation of fluoride ions which may be nephrotoxic.

(Ch. 22, A & S; Ch. 5, D)

a **True** Hyperkalaemia, a low bicarbonate concentration, and a raised urea concentration are typical of acute renal failure.

b **True** Addison's disease results in hyponatraemia, and renal failure secondary to cardiac failure.

c **False** Water retention is the main feature of inappropriate ADH secretion; serum sodium is usually lower and urea concentration is reduced.

d **False** Liver failure is associated with hypokalaemia and diminished production of urea.

e **False** A similar picture to that of inappropriate ADH secretion would be seen. (Ch. 5 A & S)

(Ch. 10, D)

a **True** This is a result of impaired aldosterone metabolism.

b **True** Impaired synthesis of albumin is a feature of liver disease.

c **True** Conjugated and unconjugated bilirubin concentration are increased in hepatocellular jaundice.

d **False** The prothrombin time is increased because of impaired synthesis of coagulation factors and decreased uptake of fat-soluble vitamins.

e **False** Hypernatraemia occurs. (See **a**)

41 Hepatitis may be transmitted by

a Cryoprecipitate.

b Fibrinogen.

c Fresh frozen plasma.

d Anti-haemophilia globulin (factor VIII).

e Purified beef gelatin.

42 Digoxin may be useful in

a Atrial flutter.

b Cardiac tamponade.

c Paroxysmal supraventricular tachycardia.

d Junctional rhythm.

e Prinzmetal angina.

43 Acute renal failure

a Is caused most commonly by acute ischaemia due to severe haemorrhage.

b May complicate the perioperative course of patients with jaundice.

c Is associated with a urine: plasma urea ratio of 2:1 if the cause is prerenal.

d Necessitates the insertion of a CVP catheter to monitor therapy.

e Frequently results in persistent anuria.

44 Ventricular ectopic beats

a May cause heart failure.

b May convert to ventricular fibrillation in the presence of myocardial infarction.

c Should always be treated.

d Are indistinguishable from atrial extrasystoles at the radial pulse.

e May be treated with lignocaine.

a **True** Cryoprecipitate may transmit hepatitis B virus. (Ch. 13, D)
b **True** Fibrinogen is obtained by cold precipitation of plasma with alcohol. Only products which have been heat-treated may be regarded as free from risk.
c **True** Fresh frozen plasma has not been heat-treated and contains many heat-labile coagulation factors.
d **True** Human AHG may transmit hepatitis, but genetically-engineered AHG is now available.
e **False** The two gelatin solutions in common use (Gelofusine and Haemaccel) are free from hepatitis B virus.

a **True** Digoxin is used to control the ventricular rate in atrial flutter.
b **False** The treatment for cardiac tamponade is relief of the tamponade at the earliest opportunity.
c **True** Digoxin may be useful in paroxysmal supraventricular tachycardia but beta-blocker or calcium channel blocking drugs are now preferred.
d **False** Digoxin is contraindicated in junctional rhythm because it may increase block at the AV node.
e **False** The usual therapy for Prinzmetal angina is administration of calcium channel blocking drugs or beta-blockers.

a **True** Oliguria occurs because of cortical vasoconstriction in response to diminished perfusion.
b **True** This is the hepatorenal syndrome.
c **False** The urine: plasma urea ratio frequently exceeds 10:1 in acute pre-renal failure.
d **True** CVP should be monitored early to permit control of intravascular resuscitation.
e **False** The urine output is sometimes normal but tubular excretory function is impaired.

a **True** There is a disturbance of stroke volume in addition to rhythm; this may cause heart failure.
b **True** After myocardial infarction, patients should be monitored, and ventricular ectopic beats treated.
c **False** Ventricular ectopic beats may be benign and occur in the normal individual.
d **True** The ECG is the only accurate means of diagnosing the origin of ectopic beats.
e **True** Lignocaine stabilises membranes and suppresses ventricular ectopics.

45   With regard to actions of drugs on the heart

a   The effects of digoxin are potentiated by administration of calcium.

b   Thiazide diuretics may precipitate digitalis toxicity.

c   Digoxin is potentiated by hypoalbuminaemia.

d   Lanatoside C is the fastest acting intravenous glycoside.

e   Lignocaine is used usually for therapy of ventricular arrhythmias.

46   Hypokalaemia may occur in the presence of

a   Metabolic acidosis.

b   Respiratory acidosis.

c   Rapid cellular uptake of glucose.

d   Anuria.

e   Extensive muscle breakdown.

47   Features of acute obstructive jaundice include

a   Increased urinary urobilinogen concentration.

b   Increased serum unconjugated bilirubin concentration.

c   Increased faecal fat.

d   A palpable gall bladder in which there would be stones.

e   Alkaline phosphatase concentration exceeding 100 K.A. units.

48   Features of acute small bowel obstruction include

a   Nausea and vomiting.

b   Central abdominal pain worsened by movement.

c   Abdominal distension.

d   Dullness to percussion in the flanks.

e   Low pitched rumbling bowel sounds.

49   An arterial plasma bicarbonate concentration of 18 mmol/litre is consistent with

a   Metabolic acidosis.

b   Compensated metabolic acidosis.

c   Compensated metabolic alkalosis.

d   Compensated respiratory alkalosis.

e   Respiratory acidosis.

(Ch. 14, A & S; Ch. 7, D)

a True The action of digoxin is mediated by calcium.

b True Secondary to hypokalaemia induced by the diuretic.
c True This may result from diminished calcium binding by albumin.
d False Lanatoside C is not available for i.v. use.
e True Lignocaine is a Class 1 anti-arrhythmic drug.

(Ch. 22, A & S)

a False Acidosis causes a shift of potassium from the intracellular to the extracellular compartment.
b False See **a**.
c True Secondary to insulin secretion which drives extracellular potassium into the intracellular compartment.
d False Hyperkalaemia occurs in renal failure.
e False Intracellular potassium is released by damaged muscle.

(Ch. 10, D)

a False There is increased excretion of conjugated bilirubin.
b False But in longstanding cases, hepatocellular failure may occur.
c True Because of impaired excretion of bile salts, fat absorption is reduced.
d False Only severe obstruction caused by pancreatic carcinoma produces this sign.
e True This is diagnostic of biliary obstruction.

(Ch. 9, D; Ch. 32, A & S)

a True There is a risk of pulmonary aspiration preoperatively.
b False Pain of simple obstruction is usually colicky in nature.
c False Distension is associated with chronic large bowel obstruction.
d False This is a sign of ascites.
e False Characteristically, bowel sounds are increased and tinkling in nature.

(Ch. 5, D; Ch. 22, A & S)

a True An excess of hydrogen ions drives the carbonic acid/bicarbonate equilibrium to the left.
b True A reduction in bicarbonate ion concentration defines metabolic acidosis.
c False A plasma bicarbonate concentration of 18 mmol/litre indicates moderate to severe metabolic acidosis.
d True Renal compensatory mechanisms excrete sodium and bicarbonate ions in respiratory alkalosis.
e False Hydrogen ion concentration and Pa_{CO_2} are increased, and HCO_3 is normal or slightly elevated.

50   **The following feature is characteristic of the accompanying cardiac abnormality**

a   Tapping apex beat in mitral incompetence.

b   Right atrial hypertrophy in mitral stenosis.

c   Collapsing pulse in aortic stenosis.
d   Diastolic murmur at the left sternal edge in aortic incompetence.
e   Cyanosis in congenital heart disease with right-to-left shunt.

51   **Diagnosis of brain-stem death in the U K requires**

a   Absence of spinal reflexes.
b   Flat EEG.
c   No ventilatory movement when Pa_{CO_2} exceeds 7 kPa.

d   No gag reflex following passage of a suction catheter down the trachea.
e   Absence of contrast medium in anterior and middle cerebral arteries on carotid angiography.

52   **In tetanus**

a   Reflex hyperactivity occurs.

b   ST and T wave changes occur in the ECG because of toxic myocarditis.
c   The relaxant of choice for IPPV is pancuronium.

d   Prognosis is independent of incubation period.
e   Tracheostomy is always indicated.

53   **Myasthenia gravis**

a   Is probably an autoimmune disease.

b   Exhibits increased sensitivity to non-depolarising and depolarising relaxants.
c   Resembles myasthenic syndrome in the response to muscle relaxants.
d   Requires thymectomy only in patients exceeding 50 years of age with a thymoma.
e   Is exacerbated by ACTH therapy before there is improvement.

(Ch. 7, D)

a False Rapid closure of the mitral valve in mitral stenosis may produce a tapping quality.
b True This may be manifest as a prominent 'a' wave in the jugular venous pulse.
c False This is characteristic of aortic incompetence.
d True Heard best during expiration with the patient leaning forward.
e True Desaturated blood reaches the systemic circulation.

(Ch. 42, A & S)

a False Spinal reflexes may occur in the absence of brain stem integrity.
b False The EEG is not required as part of the protocol in the UK.
c True The Pa_{CO_2} must be checked, or the lungs ventilated with 5% CO_2 in oxygen.
d True There should be no response to passage of a suction catheter into the nose, mouth or bronchial tree.
e False Angiography is unnecessary.

(Ch. 19, D)

a True The exotoxin has an affinity for motor nerve endings and anterior horn cells.
b False But autonomic nerve involvement may cause cardiovascular complications.
c False Hypertension may complicate the disease and this would be worsened by pancuronium.
d False The shorter the incubation period the more severe the attacks.
e False Local tetanus may affect only the muscles near the infected wound.

(Ch. 41, A & S; Ch. 15, D)

a True The number of acetylcholine receptors is diminished because of an autoimmune reaction between the receptor and an antibody.
b False The response to depolarising relaxants may be variable but is often normal.
c False There is sensitivity to all relaxants in myasthenic syndrome.
d False Thymectomy is effective in the early stages of the disease.
e True Steroid treatment is not recommended as the initial treatment.

54   Extradural haemorrhage

    a Often results from a tear in the middle meningeal artery.

    b If severe enough to cause clinical signs, causes hemiplegia initially on the same side as the haemorrhage.

    c Initially causes pupil dilation on the same side as the haemorrhage.

    d Is often followed by a lucid interval after a period of concussion.

    e Is often bilateral, in common with subdural haematomas.

---

55   Inhalation of large food particles rapidly causes

    a Cyanosis.

    b Asphyxia.

    c Mediastinal shift.

    d Pneumothorax.

    e Bronchospasm.

---

56   Concerning hip fractures in the elderly

    a Pulmonary embolus is the most common cause of death.

    b A delay of 7–10 days before surgery is beneficial.

    c Spinal anaesthesia is a useful alternative to general anaesthesia.

    d Spinal anaesthesia decreases mortality in comparison with general anaesthesia.

    e All patients are hypoxic in the immediate postoperative period, irrespective of anaesthetic technique.

---

57   In chronic bronchitis

    a There is usually a history of chronic smoke inhalation.

    b Mucus secretion is increased.

    c The ratio FEV_1/FVC is normal.

    d The ten-year survival rate is poor.

    e Residual volume (RV) is reduced.

(Ch. 15, D)

a **True** The artery is superficial and susceptible to injury.
b **False** Usually contralateral hemiplegia occurs.

c **False** Ipsilateral pupillary dilation is a late sign produced by third nerve compression.
d **True** There is a danger in discharging a patient home during this time.
e **False** Unilateral injury is more common.

(Ch. 32, A & S)

a **True** Large food particles may cause upper airway obstruction and asphyxia.
b **True** See above.
c **False** Mediastinal movement is not an early feature in the acute phase of inhalation of large particles.
d **False** Pneumothorax is unlikely in this situation.
e **True** Unsuspected aspiration of stomach contents on induction of anaesthesia or during the course of anaesthesia may precipitate bronchospasm.

(Ch. 27, Ch. 24, A & S)

a **False** Bronchopneumonia is the most common cause of death in these patients.
b **False** Although some immediate resuscitation may be required, in general the earlier the operation is performed, the better the outlook.
c **True** However, care has to be taken to avoid the hypotension which may accompany spinal anaesthesia in an emergency anaesthetic.
d **False** Although there is a significant difference in mortality in the first four weeks after surgery, there is no long-term difference following spinal or general anaesthesia.
e **False** Hypoxaemia occurs immediately after anaesthesia following the use of nitrous oxide, but not after spinal anaesthesia.

(Ch. 8, D)

a **True** Chronic bronchitis is much more common in smokers than in non-smokers.
b **True** There is overactivity of the mucus-secreting glands in the bronchi and bronchioles.
c **False** FEV_1 is reduced and the ratio of FEV_1 to forced vital capacity is also reduced.
d **False** Patients may survive for many years, though with gradually diminishing respiratory reserve.
e **False** Residual volume may be increased because of air trapping.

58 The following are associated with a low fixed cardiac output

a Aortic regurgitation.

b Aortic stenosis.
c Mitral stenosis.
d Mild hypothyroidism.

e Digoxin toxicity.

59 A patient with a longstanding paralysis caused by transection of the spinal cord at T5

a Has flaccid legs.

b Is poikilothermic.
c Has a mass autonomic reflex.

d Has a reduction in FVC.

e May demonstrate a large increase in serum K^+ concentration in response to suxamethonium.

60 The following are features of cervical sympathetic chain damage

a Enophthalmos.
b Miosis.
c Dilated conjunctival vessels.
d Congested nasal mucosa.

e Ptosis.

61 Hypothyroidism

a Is accompanied rarely by symptoms of myxoedema.
b Is complicated by ulnar nerve compression and tingling in the fingers.
c May result in difficulty with tracheal intubation because of tongue enlargement.
d Is occasionally accompanied by a pericardial effusion which is visible on X-ray.
e Results in a decrease in cardiac output.

a False The left ventricular stroke volume may be 2–3 times normal, but aortic flow may be reduced because of valvular regurgitation.
b True Restricted cardiac output may result in syncope on exercise.
c True The reduced left ventricular output may result in pulmonary oedema.
d False Basal metabolic rate is reduced, but the cardiac output although reduced is not necessarily fixed. Cardiac failure may occur in the later stages. *(Ch. 12, D)*
e False Bradycardia and coupled ventricular extrasystoles may occur.

a False With transection of the spinal cord at T5, there would be spastic paralysis.
b False The thermoregulatory centre is not affected.
c True The mass reflex comprises urination, defaecation, sweating and cardiovascular lability; it occurs in patients with chronic paraplegia
d True Loss of the use of the lower thoracic muscles in expiration results in a decrease in FVC.
e False The rise in potassium associated with suxamethonium is a transient phenomenon which occurs between approximately 24 hours and 6 months after denervation injuries. *(Ch. 41, A & S)*

a True This is a feature of Horner's syndrome.
b True This is a feature of Horner's syndrome.
c True This results from lack of sympathetically induced vasoconstriction.
d True The sympathetic supply to the nose causes vasoconstriction – thus sympathetic block or damage causes vasodilatation.
e True The levator palpebrae superioris is innervated partly by the sympathetic system, and ptosis may therefore result from damage to the sympathetic supply.

a False Myxoedema often, but not invariably, accompanies hypothyroidism.
b False Carpal tunnel compression of the median nerve is associated with hypothyroidism.
c True Tongue enlargement is a feature of hypothyroidism and may render laryngoscopy difficult.
d True Cardiomegaly and a pericardial effusion may be present. The effusion usually resolves with treatment of the hypothyroidism.
e True Cardiac output and basal metabolic rate are reduced. Drug distribution and metabolism are affected.

62 A patient with a serum Na^+ concentration of 125 mmol/litre and K^+ concentration of 6.1 mmol/litre has features compatible with

    a Hypopituitarism.

    b Addison's disease.

    c Hyperaldosteronism.

    d Cushing's syndrome.

    e Inappropriate secretion of ADH.

63 In a comatose diabetic patient, the following are more likely to be features of hypoglycaemia than ketoacidosis

    a Dry mucous membranes.

    b Extensor plantar response.

    c Hyperventilation.

    d Hypotension.

    e Sweating.

64 Warming stored blood immediately before transfusion

    a Is associated with an increased incidence of infection.

    b Increases CO_2 content.

    c Increases O_2 content.

    d Is associated with a lower incidence of arrhythmias.

    e Shifts the oxyhaemoglobin dissociation curve to the right.

65 Systemic arterial pressure may be overestimated by sphygmomanometry if

    a The cuff is too small for the arm.

    b The patient has severe arteriosclerosis.

    c The cuff is deflated very slowly.

    d The sphygmomanometer is at a higher level than the patient.

    e The patient is obese.

(Ch. 12, D)

a True Hypopituitarism leads to an Addisonian crisis because of absence of secretion of ACTH.
b True These results are characteristic of an Addisonian patient.
c False Hyperaldosteronism causes hypernatraemia and hypokalaemia – Conn's syndrome.
d False In Cushing's syndrome, there is sodium retention and loss of potassium.
e False Although increased ADH secretion results in hyponatraemia, hyperkalaemia is not a feature.

(Ch. 12, D)

a False Ketoacidosis is accompanied by dehydration which causes dry mucous membranes.
b True Brisk extensor plantar reflexes accompany hypoglycaemic coma.
c False Hyperventilation (Kussmaul's respiration) is one of the characteristic features of ketoacidosis.
d False Hypotension occurs in ketoacidosis because of loss of extracellular fluid.
e True Hypoglycaemia is associated with increased sympathoadrenal activity.

(Ch. 32, A & S)

a False There is no increased incidence of infection associated with the use of blood warmers.
b False Carriage of CO_2 is uninfluenced.
c False The solubility of oxygen in plasma decreases with increased temperature. Oxygen carriage in whole blood is unchanged.
d True Transfusion of cold blood may produce arrhythmias. Warming blood before transfusion obviates this risk.
e True The oxyhaemoglobin dissociation curve is shifted to the right by increasing temperature. *(Ch. 2, A & S)*

(Ch. 21, A & S)

a True If the cuff is too narrow the arterial pressure may be overestimated. The cuff should cover two-thirds of the length of the upper arm.
b True In this case, the pulse pressure also tends to be abnormally high. *(Ch. 7, D)*
c False The converse is true. Rapid deflation tends to result in overestimation.
d False The column of air in the tube between the patient and the mercury manometer has little influence.
e True A larger cuff than usual may be required in an obese patient.

66   **In a state of water intoxication, the following are true**

a   A low serum sodium concentration is present.

b   There may be a low urine output.

c   There is increased right atrial pressure.

d   Increased body weight is present.

e   Treatment with frusemide 80 mg is indicated.

67   **In a patient with jaundice, a serum alkaline phosphatase concentration of 300 IU/litre suggests**

a   The presence of a hepatoma.

b   Hepatocellular dysfunction.

c   Biliary obstruction.
d   Cholangitis.
e   That gamma-glutamyl transferase (γ-GT) concentration is always elevated.

68   **Raynaud's disease**

a   Responds consistently to vasodilators.

b   Affects fingers more often than toes.

c   Never causes irreversible ischaemia.

d   Presents with pain as the commonest symptom.

e   May be associated with cryoglobulinaemia.

69   **Peripheral deep vein thrombosis**

a   Is associated commonly with chronic nonmalignant medical conditions.
b   Is associated with malignancy.
c   Comprises platelet thrombus.

d   May lead to acute cor pulmonale.

e   Is associated with thrombocytopenia.

(Ch. 22, A & S; Ch. 5, D)

a True Water intoxication dilutes plasma sodium concentration and reduces plasma osmolality.

b True This may result from inappropriate secretion of ADH or renal damage.

c True Water retention causes increased ECF (and plasma) volume. Stimulation of right atrial receptors suppresses ADH secretion and causes a diuresis.

d True Weight is used frequently to monitor haemodialysis in patients with renal failure.

e False Therapy consists of treatment of the underlying cause, restricting water intake and, in severe cases, administration of 5% sodium chloride.

(Ch. 10, D)

a False Alpha-fetoprotein concentration is elevated in association with hepatoma.

b False Alkaline phosphatase concentration increases with biliary obstruction.

c True See **b**.

d True A picture of biliary obstruction is produced.

e True Elevation of gamma-glutamyl transferase concentration occurs in biliary obstruction. It is a sensitive index of liver abnormality.

(Ch. 7, D)

a False Although nifedipine may be useful, the response to vasodilators is not universally successful.

b True The disorder is usually bilateral, and fingers are affected more than toes.

c False In the later stages, ischaemic changes of the digits and gangrene may occur.

d False Numbness, tingling and burning are more common presenting features than pain.

e True Cryoglobulins occur in association with secondary Raynaud's disease or phenomenon.

(Ch. 7, D)

a False Peripheral thrombosis is not a common feature of chronic medical disease per se.

b True Increased blood coaguability may occur in malignant disease.

c False Although platelet thrombus may initiate the process, fibrin and red cells comprise the elements of the thrombus.

d True Pulmonary thromboembolism may produce acute right heart failure.

e False Increases in platelets and platelet adhesiveness are factors which promote venous thrombosis.

70   In fat embolism the following features may be present

a   Pyrexia.

b   Fat globules in the sputum.
c   Fat globules in the urine.
d   Petechiae.
e   Reduced Pa_{O_2}.

71   Pleural effusion is a common complication of

a   Staphylococcal pneumonia.

b   Streptococcal pneumonia.

c   Mycoplasma pneumonia.

d   Viral pneumonia

e   Pneumococcal pneumonia.

72   Jaundice without bilirubinuria may result from

a   Ingestion of chlorpromazine.
b   Infective hepatitis.

c   Bile duct obstruction.
d   Haemolytic anaemia.

e   Metastatic liver secondaries.

73   The insulin-dependent diabetic perioperatively

a   Must receive short-acting insulin therapy on the day before surgery to achieve stabilisation.

b   May exhibit proteinuria as a result of diabetic nephropathy.

c   Should have preoperative measurements of arterial blood pressure in the supine and erect positions.

d   Requires less insulin if blood transfusion is required.

e   May receive low-dose insulin infusion without concurrent glucose administration.

(Ch. 42, A & S)

a True Dyspnoea, cyanosis and pyrexia may occur as a result of pulmonary fat embolism.

b True

c True

d True Particularly in the upper chest, neck and conjunctivae.

e True Because of increased V/Q scatter, Pa_{O_2} may be low even in the presence of a high inspired oxygen concentration.

(Ch. 8, D)

a False Staphylococcal pneumonia may occur as a complication of influenza or as suppurative pneumonia. Pleural reaction and effusion is less common in these conditions.

b True Streptococcal pneumonia is the most common type of primary pneumonia; pleural effusion may complicate this.

c False The pneumonia of mycoplasma produces fewer clinical signs than classical pneumonia.

d False The physical signs of viral pneumonia are less marked and pleural effusion is not common.

e True Pleural effusion may complicate classical pneumococcal pneumonia.

(Ch. 10, D)

a True Chlorpromazine is hepatotoxic. *(Ch. Gui, BNF)*

b True Hepatocellular damage results in loss of conjugation of bilirubin. Only conjugated bilirubin is found in the urine, because it is water-soluble.

c False Conjugated bilirubin is available for urinary excretion.

d True Unconjugated bilirubin is the cause of jaundice in haemolytic anaemia.

e False There is a large reserve of liver function, and conjugation is maintained until a very late stage of metastatic spread.

(Ch. 41, A & S; Ch. 12, D)

a False Well-controlled diabetics on moderate doses of long-acting insulin may be managed safely on the day before surgery without changing the regimen.

b True Proteinuria signifies increasing renal failure. Accompanying hypertension should be controlled.

c True Variation between supine and erect arterial pressure may indicate the presence of autonomic neuropathy. Severe hypotension may complicate IPPV.

d False Blood transfusion and Hartmann's solution increase insulin requirements because lactate stimulates gluconeogenesis.

e True Whilst this may be adequate for minor surgery of short duration, insulin and glucose combinations are usually prescribed.

74 **An i.v. infusion of dopamine 10 µg/kg per minute produces an increase in**

a Cardiac output.

b Renal blood flow.

c Systemic vascular resistance.
d Urine output.

e Urinary sodium excretion.

75 **Fluid overload may cause**

a An increase in urine output.
b An increase in CVP.
c Increased lung compliance.

d Dependent oedema.
e Hepatojugular reflux.

76 **A young female patient with a history of asthma presents for minor surgery under general anaesthesia**

a A history of atopy and allergy are likely.
b High pitched inspiratory rhonchi would be heard on auscultation of the chest.
c Perioperative steroid cover should be given if the patient has received steroids in the previous six months.

d Halothane is the preferred volatile agent.
e High concentrations of oxygen are safe if administered postoperatively.

77 **The following drugs instilled into the conjunctival sac cause mydriasis**

a Ephedrine.

b Timolol.

c Amethocaine.
d Homatropine.
e Cocaine.

(Ch. 13, A & S; Appx. IV (b), A & S)

a True Dopamine in this dose has a positive inotropic effect but causes little or no peripheral vasoconstriction.
b True Reduction in renal arterial resistance results in increased renal blood flow and glomerular filtration rate.
c False There is little or no peripheral vasoconstrictor effect in this dose.
d True An increase in urine output occurs as a result of the renal and inotropic effects of dopamine.
e True Increases in renal blood flow, glomerular filtration rate and sodium excretion occur at low and medium doses of dopamine.

(Ch. 4, Ch. 22, A & S)

a True This is the normal physiological method of fluid regulation.
b True Fluid overload leads to an increase in central venous pressure.
c False A decrease in lung compliance occurs with pulmonary oedema secondary to fluid overload.
d True Dependent oedema is a sign of fluid overload.
e True When venous pressure is increased transiently by pressure on the abdomen, the level of pulsation moves upwards in the neck – hepatojugular reflux. *(Ch. 7, D)*

(Ch. 8, D)

a True 'Early onset' asthma occurs more commonly in atopic individuals.
b False Prolonged expiration and expiratory rhonchi are the hallmarks of asthma.
c False For minor surgery in a patient not taking steroids, this is unnecessary. However, close postoperative supervision is essential and steroid treatment should be considered if symptoms dictate.
d True Halothane possesses bronchodilator properties.
e True There is no loss of central CO_2 response in patients with asthma alone.

---

a True This is caused by stimulation of the beta-adrenoceptors in the dilator pupillae. *(Ch. 13, A & S)*
b False Timolol causes pupillary constriction and is used in the treatment of glaucoma. *(Ch. 11, BNF)*
c False Amethocaine is a local anaesthetic.
d True Homatropine is a shorter acting mydriatic than atropine.
e True Cocaine has sympathomimetic actions. *(Ch. 15, A & S)*

78   Chronic adrenal insufficiency leads to

a   Hyponatraemia.
b   Hypokalaemia.
c   Hypovolaemia.
d   Hypotension.

e   Hypoglycaemia.

79   The following may be features of acute myocardial infarction

a   Basal crepitations.

b   Epigastric pain.

c   Absence of pain.
d   Effective pain relief with glyceryl trinitrate.
e   Dyspnoea.

80   Abnormal patterns may occur in lead V_5 of the ECG in

a   Anterior mural ischaemia.
b   Lateral wall ischaemia.
c   Inferior ventricular ischaemia.
d   Posterior ventricular ischaemia.
e   Transmural infarct.

81   After cardiac arrest following acute myocardial infarction (MI):

a   Lignocaine is indicated for prevention of atrial tachycardia.

b   Oxygen should be given by mask or nasal prongs.
c   Defibrillation is likely to be effective.

d $NaHCO_3$ 200 mmol is indicated.
e $NaHCO_3$ 1 mmol/kg is recommended.

(Ch. 12, D; Ch. 22, A & S)

a True   Because of absence of mineralocorticoid activity.
b False   Hyperkalaemia occurs in Addison's disease.
c True   This occurs because of excess sodium and water losses.
d True   Hypotension accompanies hypovolaemia. Normal reflex maintenance of arterial pressure is impaired also, and postural hypotension may be particularly troublesome.
e True   Reactive hypoglycaemia may occur after a carbohydrate meal. Cortisol is one of the physiological antagonists to insulin.

(Ch. 7, D; Ch. 19, A & S)

a True   Basal crepitations signify left ventricular failure which may complicate acute myocardial infarction.
b True   The pain of acute myocardial infarction may be perceived in the epigastrium.
c True   Myocardial infarction may be painless.
d False   GTN does not relieve the pain of acute myocardial infarction.
e True   'Cardiac asthma' (acute left ventricular failure) may be associated with acute myocardial infarction.

(Ch. 7, D)

a False   Changes occur in leads V_2-V_4.
b True   Left sided chest leads reflect lateral ischaemic changes.
c False   Leads II, III, and aVF usually show inferior ischaemia.
d False   Changes would be seen only in leads V_1 and V_4.
e True   Q waves would be present in a lateral transmural infarction.

(Ch. 44, A & S; Ch. 7, D)

a False   Lignocaine may be indicated to prevent recurrence of ventricular fibrillation.
b True   Gas transfer may be impaired and the patient may be hypotensive.
c True   Cardiac arrest after acute MI is likely to be caused by ventricular fibrillation. This is more common than asystole.
d False   In the absence of metabolic acidosis, bicarbonate is not indicated.
e False   Bicarbonate adds a significant sodium load and increases Pa_{CO_2}.

82 The following arrhythmias in an adult are treated in the acute situation by the accompanying therapy

  a Sinus bradycardia – atropine 0.6 mg i.v.
  b Ventricular tachycardia – lignocaine 100 mg i.v.

  c Asystole – adrenaline 0.05 mg i.v.
  d Atrial flutter – cardioversion.

  e Sinus tachycardia – verapamil 5 mg i.v.

83 The following are not associated with increased water loss

  a Diabetes insipidus.
  b Acute tubular necrosis.
  c Strenuous exercise.

  d Inappropriate secretion of antidiuretic hormone (ADH).
  e Treatment with carbonic anhydrase inhibitors.

84 The following are indicated in the management of a patient who has taken an overdose of tricyclic antidepressants

  a Immediate i.v. administration of a beta-blocker.

  b Measurement of serum tricyclic concentration.

  c Forced acid diuresis.
  d Diazepam.

  e Pyridostigmine.

85 With respect to carbon monoxide poisoning

  a Infants are at greater risk than adults.
  b Toxicity occurs at carboxyhaemoglobin concentrations less than 5%.
  c Cardiorespiratory arrest may occur.
  d Toxicity never occurs with inhalation of natural gas.

  e Hyperbaric oxygen treatment is useful.

(Ch. 14, Ch. 44, A & S)

a True Atropine is an antimuscarinic.
b True The membrane-stabilising action of lignocaine is appropriate for ventricular arrythymias.
c False 1 mg (1000 µg) is appropriate.
d True Cardioversion is the most appropriate initial treatment. Digoxin is second line therapy.
e False Verapamil is not the agent of first choice for sinus tachycardia. A beta-blocker such as metoprolol might be appropriate treatment if carotid sinus massage fails.

(Ch. 22, Ch. 14, A & S; Ch. 5, D)

a False Diabetes is associated classically with water loss.
b True Oliguria is a normal feature of acute tubular necrosis.
c False During severe exercise, sweating may deplete total body water by several litres.
d True ADH produces water retention.
e False Carbonic anhydrase inhibitors act as diuretic agents.

(Ch. 17, D; Ch. Em, BNF)

a False Tachyarrhythmias associated with tricyclic overdose are treated most appropriately with physostigmine.
b False There is no indication for measuring tricyclic concentrations in the treatment of poisoning.
c False Forced acid diuresis is an inappropriate therapy.
d True Diazepam may be used to reduce cerebral irritability which is a feature in some patients.
e False Pyridostigmine has weak antimuscarinic effects and does not cross the blood/brain barrier.

(p. 1104, D [10th ed])

a True
b False Carboxyhaemoglobin concentrations of up to 5% have been recorded in cigarette smokers. *(Ch. 2, A & S)*
c True Failure of oxygen delivery to the tissues results in hypoxaemia.
d True There is no carbon monoxide in natural gas. However, carbon monoxide may be released if there is incomplete combustion of natural gas.
e True Hyperbaric oxygen increases the rate of elimination of carbon monoxide.

86   In paracetamol overdosage

a   Coma is uncommon.
b   Hypoglycaemia is a danger.
c   Prothrombin time may increase.
d   Haemofiltration is a useful measure.

e   N-acetylcysteine therapy is indicated.

87   A pulmonary artery catheter may be used

a   To assess left atrial pressure.

b   To diagnose pulmonary hypertension.

c   To measure left ventricular output.

d   Only via the internal jugular vein.

e   With a dye dilution technique to measure cardiac output.

88   In carcinoma of the head of the pancreas

a   Painless jaundice is a common feature.
b   Preoperative glucose tolerance testing is indicated.

c   Serum acid phosphatase concentration is increased.

d   Perioperative treatment with mannitol is indicated.

e   The one-year survival is less than 10%.

89   Dextran

a   Affects coagulation.

b   Is allergenic.

c   Causes rouleaux formation if mixed with blood.

d   May cause renal damage.
e   May interfere with cross-matching.

(Ch. 17, D; Ch. Em, BNF)

a True   Coma is not a common feature of paracetamol overdose
b True   This may occur after an interval of approximately 36 h.
c True   Because of inhibition of synthesis secondary to hepatic damage.
d False   Haemofiltration is not indicated. However, haemoperfusion and/or haemodialysis may be indicated in the presence of liver or renal failure.
e True   N-acetylcysteine and methionine may protect the liver if given within 10–12 h of ingestion of paracetamol

---

(Ch. 21, A & S)

a True   Pulmonary capillary wedge pressure is related to left atrial pressure and may be measured with this device.
b True   Pulmonary artery pressure may be measured (normally 25/10 mmHg).
c True   A thermodilution catheter may be used to measure the output of the right ventricle which is equal (within 1%) to the left ventricular output.
d False   Any large vein will suffice, although the internal jugular vein is convenient.
e False   Thermodilution is the technique usually employed. A pulmonary artery catheter cannot be used alone to measure cardiac output by dye dilution; peripheral blood sampling is required also.

(Ch. 9, D)

a True
b True   An abnormal glucose tolerance test may be encountered preoperatively in a patient in whom this diagnosis is suspected.
c False   Serum alkaline phosphatase is increased in carcinoma of head of pancreas.
d True   Perioperative administration of mannitol is thought to decrease the likelihood of the hepatorenal syndrome developing.
e True   The prognosis is very poor.

(Ch. 9, BNF; Ch. 7 A & S)

a True   Dextran has been used for its anticoagulant properties in prevention of deep vein thrombosis.
b True   The incidence of hypersensitivity reactions to i.v. administration of Dextran is approximately 0.3%.
c True   Formation of rouleaux after mixing with blood interferes with cross-matching.
d True   Dextran 40 has been implicated in renal damage.
e True   (see **c**).

90   CPD blood which has been stored for 21 days

    a   Is rich in platelets.

    b   Has a normal 2, 3-diphosphoglycerate concentration.

    c   Has a high lactate concentration.

    d   Has a high extracellular K^+ concentration.

    e   Contains extracellular haemoglobin.

91   In chronic obstructive airways disease, a pink puffer differs from a blue bloater in having a lower.

    a FEV_1.

    b   Number of red blood cells.

    c   Base excess.

    d   FRC.

    e Pa_{O_2}.

92   An increased serum concentration of alkaline phosphatase is found in the following

    a   Obstructive jaundice.

    b   Paget's disease.

    c   Osteoporosis.

    d   Haemolytic anaemia.

    e   Prostatic carcinoma.

93   Peripheral nerve injury is likely to occur in

    a   Mid-forearm fracture involving both bones.

    b   A midshaft fracture of the humerus.

    c   Dislocated shoulder.

    d   The lithotomy position.

    e   Midshaft fracture of the femur.

(Ch. 7, Ch. 32, A & S)

a False Platelet numbers and function deteriorate after 24 hours of storage.
b False There is 20% loss of 2, 3–DPG after two weeks' storage. Levels are not restored to normal until 24 hours after transfusion.
c True The presence of high concentrations of lactic acid contributes to the low pH of stored blood.
d True Extracellular potassium concentration may be considerably higher than that of normal blood – up to 25 mmol/litre.
e True Haemolysis in vitro results in an increase in extracellular haemoglobin concentration.

(Ch. 8, D; Ch. 41, A & S)

a False In both groups of chronic obstructive airways disease, the FEV_1 is reduced.
b True In chronic hypoxaemia and type 2 respiratory failure, polycythaemia may supervene.
c True Hypercapnia produces a compensatory non-respiratory alkalosis.
d False In emphysema, destruction of lung tissue and increase in the anteroposterior diameter of the chest increase FRC.
e False Hypoxaemia characterises the bronchitic blue bloater.

(Ch. 10, D)

a True Increased serum alkaline phosphatase concentration is a feature of obstructive jaundice.
b True This is caused by osteoblastic activity. *(Ch. 14, D)*
c False Osteoblastic activity is not a feature of osteoporosis.
d False Haemolytic activity itself does not result in alterations in serum alkaline phosphatase concentration.
e False This is associated classically with an increased acid phosphatase concentration, but secondary prostatic carcinoma may be associated with increased alkaline phosphatase concentration.

a False The median and ulnar nerves are more vulnerable with wrist and elbow injuries.
b True The radial nerve may be involved in a midshaft humeral fracture.
c True The cords of the brachial plexus lie in close proximity and may be involved in shoulder dislocations. *(Ch. 26 A & S)*
d True A misplaced leg support may result in compression of the lateral popliteal nerve. *(Ch. 20, A & S)*
e False The femoral nerve branches proximal to the midshaft of the femur. The sciatic nerve is well protected by muscles.

94   In chronic anaemia (Hb < 5 g /dl), the patient compensates with

a   Increased cardiac output.
b   Decreased blood volume.

c   Hyperventilation at rest.

d   Shift of the oxyhaemoglobin dissociation curve (ODC) to the left.
e   Decrease in red cell 2, 3-DPG concentration.

---

95   A low serum sodium concentration accompanied by low total body sodium content occurs in

a   Heart failure with oedema.

b   Renal failure.
c   Liver failure.

d   Water intoxication.

e   Addison's disease.

---

96   Pulmonary fibrosis

a   Complicates bronchiectasis.
b   Results in an increase in pulmonary compliance.
c   May supervene in chronic mitral valve disease.

d   Produces a restrictive defect in lung function tests.
e   May occur following treatment with bleomycin.

---

97   Tumours associated with a low serum potassium concentration include

a   Chondrosarcoma.
b   Acoustic neuroma.
c   Carcinoid.

d   Villous papilloma of the rectum.
e   Phaeochromocytoma.

(Ch. 7, A & S)

a **True** Both stroke volume and heart rate increase.
b **False** With a chronic reduction in red cell mass, there is an accompanying increase in plasma volume; blood volume is unchanged.
c **False** The clinical features of chronic anaemia reflect the diminished oxygen carrying capacity of the blood. Hyperventilation is not present at rest, but there is dyspnoea on exertion. *(Ch. 13, D)*
d **False** The ODC is shifted to the right in chronic anaemia (vide infra).
e **False** There is increased synthesis of 2, 3-DPG which is responsible for the shift of the ODC to the right.

(Ch. 22, A & S; Ch. 5, D)

a **False** Sodium retention secondary to aldosterone secretion is common in heart failure. *(Ch. 7, D)*
b **False** A low total body sodium does not accompany renal failure.
c **False** Sodium retention occurs because of impaired aldosterone metabolism. *(Ch. 10, D)*
d **False** Isolated water intoxication results from water retention in the presence of a normal total body sodium.
e **True** But serum cortisol concentration should be determined to make the diagnosis. *(Ch. 10, D)*

(Ch. 8, D)

a **True** 'Replacement' fibrosis is associated with bronchiectasis.
b **False** Increased stiffness of the lungs accounts for decreased compliance.
c **True** Pulmonary oedema becomes chronic, and interstitial fibrosis may follow.
d **True** Both FEV_1 and FVC are reduced.
e **True**

---

a **False** Hypokalaemia is not a recognised feature. *(Ch. 14, D)*
b **False** This is not a recognised feature. *(Ch. 15, D)*
c **True** Diarrhoea is a feature of carcinoid syndrome, and electrolyte imbalance may occur. *(Ch. 36, A & S)*
d **True** This tumour is associated classically with potassium loss.
e **False** Phaeochromocytoma is a catecholamine-secreting tumour and is not associated with hypokalaemia.

98   P waves are absent from the ECG in

a   Atrial fibrillation.
b   Ventricular tachycardia.

c   Massive pulmonary embolism.

d   First degree heart block.

e   Nodal rhythm.

99   Tetany occurs in

a   Anoxia.
b   Hypercalcaemia.
c   Hypokalaemia.

d   Alkalosis.

e   *Cl. welchii* infection.

100   An increased Pa_{CO_2} is found in the following

a   Those living at altitude.
b   Obstructive sleep apnoea.

c   Early septicaemia.

d   Acidosis from renal causes.

e   During infusion of bicarbonate.

a True The fibrillary waves of atrial fibrillation do not constitute P waves.

b True In ventricular tachycardia, there is no time for automatic depolarisation of the atria, and any atrial depolarisation which occurs retrogradely is hidden in the ventricular waves.

c False P waves should not normally be absent with massive pulmonary embolism, unless asystole occurs.

d False In first degree heart block, the interval from the beginning of the P wave to the beginning of the R wave exceeds 0.2 s.

e True In nodal rhythm, ventricular depolarisation is initiated at the atrio-ventricular node; it is impossible to detect P waves, as they occur synchronously with ventricular depolarisation and are hidden in the QRS complex.

(Ch. 12, D)

a False This is not a feature of anoxia.

b False Tetany is a feature of hypocalcaemia.

c False Hypokalaemia causes muscle flaccidity and cardiac arrhythmias. *(Ch. 22, A & S)*

d True Alkalosis reduces the serum concentration of ionised calcium; this causes tetany and a positive Chvostek's sign.

e False This is the causative organism of tetanus.

(Ch. 2, A & S)

a False Hyperventilation occurs during adaptation to altitude. *(Ch. 20, D)*

b True Hypoventilation occurs during episodes of obstructive sleep apnoea. This is common in the early postoperative period. *(Ch. 24, A & S)*

c False Early septicaemia is accompanied usually by hyperventilation. *(Ch. 42, A & S)*

d False Respiratory compensation for metabolic acidosis results in a decreased Pa_{CO_2}.

e True Bicarbonate forms an equilibrium with carbonic acid which dissociates to carbon dioxide and water. A transient increase in Pa_{CO_2} occurs after infusion of bicarbonate.

4. Anaesthesia

1   **A 70-year-old patient presents for gastrectomy. Preoperatively, Pa_{O_2}
     is 10.5 kPa on air. 15 minutes postoperatively, the patient is awake,
     breathing oxygen 3 litre/min via nasal cannulae. Pa_{O_2} is 8 kPa, Pa_{CO_2}
     is 7 kPa. The following may be responsibe for the abnormalities**

   a   Reduced alveolar ventilation.
   b   Diffusion hypoxia.

   c   Decreased shunt.
   d   Disturbed ventilation/perfusion ratio.

   e   Depression of ventilation.

2   **The Bain system**
   a   Is suitable for infants.

   b   Is also a Mapleson C system.
   c   Fresh gas flow occurs through the outer tubing.

   d   Disconnection at the machine end causes increased dead space.
   e   Requires fresh gas flow rate > 2.5 times the minute volume with
      spontaneous ventilation to prevent rebreathing of carbon
      dioxide.

(Ch.24, A & S)

a **True** The Pa_{CO_2} is elevated.
b **False** Diffusion hypoxia is transient and is treated effectively by oxygen therapy.
c **False** Shunting is likely to be increased.
d **True** This is present during anaesthesia and may persist into the early postoperative period.
e **True** The action of respiratory depressant drugs given intraoperatively may persist into the postoperative period.

(Ch. 17, A & S)

a **False** The system is not recommended for patients less than 25 kg in weight.
b **False** It is an example of Mapleson D system.
c **False** The inner tube delivers fresh gas, and its attachment to the proximal end must be ensured before use of the system.
d **True** The outer expiratory limb forms the extra dead space.
e **True** But it is more economical with IPPV.

3   The Blease-Manley ventilator

 a   Is a minute volume divider.
 b   Is a constant flow generator.

 c   Is time cycled.

 d   Is suitable for IPPV in the asthmatic.

 e   May cause rotameter inaccuracy.

4   A successful stellate ganglion block results in

 a   Pupillary dilation.
 b   Ptosis.
 c   Hyperhidrosis of the face.
 d   Warm upper extremity.
 e   Anaesthesia of the supraglottic part of the larynx.

5   In the supraclavicular approach to brachial plexus block, the following are true

 a   The arm should be abducted to 90 degrees.
 b   The clavicle should be depressed.
 c   The needle should pass in front of the subclavian artery.
 d   Paraesthesiae in the little finger indicate that the needle is near the ulnar nerve.
 e   Phrenic nerve paralysis cannot occur.

6   Intercostal block of one rib at the posterior angle causes

 a   Somatic anaesthesia throughout the dermatome.

 b   Visceral anaesthesia.
 c   Low arterial blood pressure due to preganglionic sympathetic block.
 d   A risk of toxic blood concentrations of local anaesthetic.

 e   Vasoconstriction in the area supplied.

a True The fresh gas flow is divided into preset tidal volumes.
b False Constant flow cannot be generated by its relatively low working pressure.
c True Both between inspiration and expiration, and between expiration and inspiration. The timing is determined by the fresh gas flow rate and the tidal volume, and is changed if either parameter is altered.
d False High inflation pressures may be required in those with bronchospasm.
e True This is due to back pressure in the machine and causes the rotameter to be under-read, but newer anaesthetic machines have a device to minimise this effect.

(Ch. 43, Ch. 13, A & S)

a False This would be a manifestation of sympathetic stimulation.
b True
c False Sympathetic blockade results in inhibition of sweating.
d True Due to relaxation of sympathetic vasoconstrictor tone.
e False Sensory innervation is via the Xth cranial nerve. *(Ch. 1, A & S)*

(Ch. 26, A & S)

a False This is the position for the axillary approach to the brachial plexus.
b True Ask the patient to touch the outside of his thigh.
c False In this position, the needle would pierce the subclavian vein.
d False The ulnar nerve is formed more distally.

e False Proximal spread of local anaesthetic solution may involve the phrenic nerve.

(Ch. 26, A & S)

a False The posterior root may not be blocked, and anteriorly there is some crossover from the contralateral nerve.
b False The intercostal nerve innervates the body wall only.
c False Spread to the sympathetic chain is extremely unlikely.

d False The area is very vascular and rapid absorption of the solution occurs. With the volume used normally, there is little risk of toxicity. However, there is a risk if several intercostal nerves are blocked, and local anaesthetic solutions containing adrenaline are recommended to reduce the risk.
e False There is normally no direct effect on sympathetic fibres unless a large volume of injectate tracks into the paravertebral space. This would result in vasodilatation.

7   Hypotension during subarachnoid block may be due to

   a   Preganglionic autonomic blockade.
   b   Venoconstriction.
   c   Block of the dorsal roots.
   d   Stimulation of the vasomotor centre.

   e   Block of nerves to the adrenal medulla.

8   The volume displacement of a strain gauge pressure transducer

   a   Indicates the amount of liquid needed to fill it.

   b   Depends on the volume of the chamber.
   c   Depends on the stiffness of the diaphragm.
   d   Depends on the frequency response of the system.
   e   Is pressure dependent.

9   Halothane concentrations can be measured by

   a   Absorption of ultraviolet radiation.
   b   Infrared absorption.
   c   A Rayleigh refractometer.
   d   Changes in the elasticity of silicone rubber.
   e   The Clark electrode.

10   Fuel cell analysers can be used for

   a   Oxygen analysis.
   b CO_2 analysis.
   c   Measurement of oxygen percentage in inspired gas.

   d   Measurement of humidity.
   e   Breath-by-breath analysis of inspired gas.

11   Pressure gauges

   a   May employ the Bourdon principle.
   b   Can be used to measure gas flow.

   c   Can regulate gas pressure.

   d   Can be used to measure temperature.

   e   Indicate absolute pressure.

a **True** The dermatomal level of sympathetic blockade is higher than that of analgesia.
b **False** Sympathetic blockade produces vasodilatation.
c **False** The dorsal roots carry afferent information only.
d **False** The brain stem vasomotor centre is unaffected unless the block is extremely high!
e **True** This is a contributory element in the genesis of hypotension.

a **False** A continuous column of liquid is needed between the patient and the transducer, but this volume is unrelated to the volume displacement of the transducer.
b **False**
c **True** A stiff diaphragm is displaced to a lesser extent.
d **True** At resonant frequency, volume displacement is increased.
e **True**

a **True** This is the principle of the Dräger narkotest halothane meter.
b **True**
c **True** This may be used to calibrate vaporisers.
d **True** This is a characteristic of halothane.
e **False** This measures oxygen concentration.

a **True** The galvanic cell generates current proportional to oxygen partial pressure.
b **False**
c **True** The partial pressure is measured. Back pressure influences the displayed concentration.
d **False** Humidity does not affect the reading.
e **False** The response time is too slow for breath-by-breath analysis.

a **True** A coiled metal tube responds to differences in pressure.
b **True** Provided flow is laminar, pressure gradient is directly proportional to flow rate.
c **False** A pressure-reducing valve, which is more correctly termed a pressure-regulating valve, performs this task.
d **True** As temperature is proportional to pressure of a gas, this is theoretically possible.
e **False** Pressure gauges indicate gauge pressure.

12   During one lung anaesthesia in the lateral position, Pa_{O_2} depends upon

a   Inspired O_2.

b   Cardiac output.

c   Perfusion of the unventilated lung.
d   Haematocrit.

e   Mixed venous P_{O_2}.

---

13   A 15-year-old child, whose brother died following an anaesthetic having developed a high temperature, presents for elective surgery. The following should be performed in addition to normal investigations.

a   Muscle biopsy.

b   Serum sodium concentration.
c   Creatinine phosphokinase concentration.
d   Cholinesterase concentration.
e   Urinalysis.

---

14   The following are associated with increased intracolonic pressure

a N_2O anaesthesia.
b   Morphine.

c   Neostigmine.
d   Adrenaline.

e   An epidural to T6.

(Ch. 39, A & S)

a True Because of intrapulmonary shunting, at least 40% inspired oxygen is required usually to achieve a normal Pa_{O_2}.

b True Low cardiac output may increase arterial P_{O_2} if it causes reduced pulmonary artery pressure, resulting in decreased perfusion of the upper, unventilated lung. However, the arteriovenous oxygen content difference is increased by a reduction in cardiac output, and for a given shunt fraction, arterial P_{O_2} is decreased.

c True Perfusion of the lungs varies with pulmonary artery pressure (see **b**).

d True Decreased haematocrit may decrease oxygen delivery to the tissues, change A–V content difference, and, for a given cardiac output and shunt fraction, affect Pa_{O_2}.

e True

(Ch. 23, A & S)

a True The possibility of malignant hyperpyrexia should be entertained, and this test is specific.

b False

c False This test is insensitive.

d False **b**, **c** and **d** are unhelpful in the diagnosis of MH.

e False This should be part of routine preoperative screening in any patient.

a True Nitrous oxide diffuses into air-filled body cavities. *(Ch. 9, A & S)*

b True Because of increase in non-propulsive smooth muscle activity of the gut. *(Ch. 11, A & S)*

c True This is mediated via activity in the parasympathetic end organ.

d False Sympathetic stimulation reduces splanchnic vascularity and activity. *(Ch. 13, A & S)*

e True The gut is contracted due to unopposed vagal activity. *(Ch. 26, A & S)*

15   The following predispose to regurgitation of gastric contents into the pharynx.

a   Hiatus hernia.

b   Raised intragastric pressure.
c   Induction in lithotomy position.

d   Head-down left lateral position.
e   Cricoid pressure.

16   Junctional rhythm occurring during anaesthesia

a   Is usually irregular.

b   Has an abnormal QRS complex.

c   Leads to a reduction in arterial pressure requiring treatment.

d   May be treated with i.v. atropine.
e   Is associated with the use of halothane.

17   The following are generally accepted methods used to reduce suxamethonium muscle pain

a   Deepening anaesthesia before use.

b   A prior small dose of gallamine.

c   A prior small dose of suxamethonium.

d   Concurrent use of morphine.

e   Administration by infusion.

18   During anaesthesia, signs of mismatched transfusion include

a   Raised arterial pressure.
b   Apnoea.
c   Oozing.

d   Haematuria.
e   Conjunctival petechiae.

a **True** Measures to reduce the acidity and volume of gastric contents should be taken in such patients.
b **True** Compression due to the gravid uterus causes this.
c **True** The gravitational effect of abdominal contents on the stomach is greater in the lithotomy position.
d **False** But if regurgitation occurs, aspiration is less likely in this position.
e **False** But pressure must be maintained to occlude the oesophagus.

a **False** The junctional node depolarises in a regular manner but more slowly than the SA node.
b **False** QRS depolarisation takes place via the normal pathway and is therefore of normal configuration.
c **False** But if hypovolaemia is allowed to exist, arterial pressure may decrease.
d **True** When treatment is required i.v. anticholinergic therapy is effective.
e **True** Halothane depresses automaticity of the SA node and nodal arrhythmias are a common accompaniment of halothane anaesthesia.

a **False** Deep anaesthesia before administration of suxamethonium has not been shown to reduce suxamethonium-related muscle pains.
b **True** The dose of gallamine needed is small – approximately 1/10th of that used to establish neuromuscular block.
c **True** The administration of a small dose of suxamethonium (0.1 mg/kg) has been described to reduce the pain from subsequent administration of suxamethonium.
d **False** Morphine and other opioids have not been shown to reduce suxamethonium muscle pain.
e **True** The administration of suxamethonium by infusion is generally accepted as reducing the incidence of suxamethonium pain.

a **False** Hypotension is usual.
b **False** Tachypnoea may occur in a spontaneously ventilating patient.
c **True** This may be an early sign of mismatched transfusion and is due to consumption coagulopathy.
d **True** Due to red cell destruction.
e **False** This is a sign typical of fat embolus.

19 **During prolonged operations, core temperature can be monitored accurately at**

a   Tympanic membrane.
b   Lower third of oesophagus.
c   Muscle in thigh.
d   Nasopharynx.
e   Pulmonary vein.

20 **The following are true of compressed medical gases**

a   Oxygen is normally stored at a pressure of 800 kPa.

b   Nitrous oxide is stored in cylinders at a pressure of 400 kPa.

c   Nitrous oxide cylinders are filled completely with liquid by the manufacturers.

d   They are stored in cylinders of molybdenum steel.

e   The amount of oxygen in a cylinder may be determined by weighing.

21 **During anaesthesia, a patient with Parkinson's disease treated with levodopa should not receive**

a   Enflurane.
b   Fentanyl.
c   Morphine.
d   Droperidol.

e   Nitrous oxide.

22 **Oliguria postoperatively is associated with**

a   Methoxyflurane anaesthesia.
b   Low cardiac output.

c   Hypothermia.
d   Hypoglycaemia.
e   Hypovolaemia.

(Ch. 21, A & S)

a True   This is used as an index of brain temperature.
b True   This reflects heart temperature. *(Ch. 18, A & S).*
c False   Muscle temperature may be influenced by the state of peripheral circulation.
d True   The probe must be in contact with the pharyngeal mucosa.
e False   The pulmonary vein is not cannulated for monitoring purposes.

(Ch. 17, A & S)

a False   Oxygen *may* be stored safely at this pressure, but the usual pressure of a full oxygen cylinder is 13.7 MPa; the pressure in pipeline delivery systems is 400 kPa.
b False   Nitrous oxide *can* be stored at 400 kPa, the pipeline pressure. However, the pressure in a full nitrous oxide cylinder is 4.4 MPa.
c False   The normal 'filling ratio' of a nitrous oxide cylinder is 0.67, this is related to the weight of nitrous oxide/weight of water to fill the cylinder. If it was full, the liquid would expand as the temperature rises with a catastrophic increase in pressure. *(Ch. 16, A & S).*
d True   These cylinders offer an acceptable compromise between strength and weight.
e False   Strictly, the amount of oxygen in a cylinder can be determined by weighing and by reference to the tare (empty) weight of the cylinder. However, as the oxygen is present as compressed gas, the change in weight is very small as the cylinder empties and this method is not of practical value.

(Ch. 15, D)

a False   Enflurane is not contraindicated.
b False   There is no contraindication to the use of fentanyl.
c False   Morphine is not contraindicated.
d True   Extrapyramidal side-effects of droperidol are commonly observed. It is a DOPA antagonist. *(Ch. 4, BNF)*
e False   Nitrous oxide is not contraindicated.

(Ch. 24, A & S)

a False   Methoxyflurane toxicity is associated with polyuria.
b True   Low cardiac output results in decreased renal blood flow. Acute tubular necrosis may occur.
c False   Hypothermia per se would not lead to oliguria.
d False   Oliguria would not result from hypoglycaemia.
e True   Hypovolaemia leads to decreased cardiac output and increased secretion of ADH.

23 **The following give an early and reliable indication of the occurrence of air embolism**

a ECG.
b BP monitoring.
c End-tidal CO_2.

d Doppler ultrasound.
e Oesophageal auscultation.

24 **With regard to transplacental passage of drugs**

a The placenta is an effective barrier.
b Fetal bradycardia may occur after epidural injection of local anaesthetics.

c Highly protein-bound drugs are transferred less.

d Amide-linked local anaesthetic drugs should be avoided.

e Fetal bradycardia is related directly to fetal blood concentrations of local anaesthetic.

25 **During epidural anaesthesia for Caesarean section**

a Never give more than 20 ml of 0.5% bupivacaine.

b The block must extend from T5 to S1.

c Syntocinon rather than ergometrine should be used.
d A paracervical block must also be performed.
e The circulation should be preloaded with Hartmann's solution.

a False ECG changes are a very late sign.
b False This is not a reliable indicator of air embolism.
c True End-tidal carbon dioxide concentration decreases due to decreased perfusion of alveoli.
d True This is an extremely sensitive method of detection of air emboli.
e False The classical mill-wheel murmur is heard late and only with a large volume of air. *(Ch. 18, A & S)*

(Ch. 6, Ch. 33, A & S)

a False Lipid-soluble drugs cross the placenta readily.
b True Toxic concentrations cross the placenta. Acceptable maternal concentrations may produce much larger fetal concentrations because of the relatively acid state of the fetal environment.
c False The free drug concentration determines the amount of placental transfer.
d False Bupivacaine and lignocaine are both acceptable agents in obstetric analgesia.
e True

(Ch. 33, A & S)

a False The maximum recommended dose of bupivacaine 0.5% is 20 ml. However, a single dose of up to 150 mg of bupivacaine (30 ml of 0.5% solution) is permissible for appropriate patients.
b False A block to S5 is necessary for adequate analgesia for Caesarean section.
c True Syntocinon provokes less nausea than does ergometrine.
d False Properly conducted epidural block is sufficient.
e True Up to 1000 ml of Hartmann's solution has been recommended as a preload for epidural Caesarean sections, but colloid solutions may be preferable if larger volumes are required.

26 **You are asked to provide anaesthesia for a patient with a breech delivery when difficulty is being experienced with the fetal head. The following are acceptable techniques**

 a Spinal.

 b Epidural.
 c Cyclopropane.

 d Thiopentone, suxamethonium, rapid sequence tracheal intubation.
 e Ketamine.

27 **Coeliac plexus block**
 a May relieve abdominal visceral pain.
 b May relieve pain of acute pancreatitis.

 c Cannot be performed without X-ray control.

 d May cause profound hypotension.
 e The tip of the needle should lie at the level of L1.

28 **Block of the trigeminal ganglion is associated with anaesthesia of**
 a Alae nasi.
 b Lower lip.
 c Angle of mandible.

 d Soft palate.
 e Eardrum.

29 **If 50% nitrous oxide is inhaled for three days**
 a The lymphocyte count falls.

 b Methionine synthetase activity is reduced.
 c Megaloblastic bone marrow changes occur.
 d B_{12} deficiency anaemia develops.

 e Peripheral neuropathy develops.

a False Unless the anaesthetist is very experienced at subarachnoid techniques, this would be inappropriate.
b False Onset time would be much too long.
c False Unless the anaesthetist is familiar with the use of cyclopropane this is inappropriate.
d True A rapid sequence induction with a familiar technique is indicated.

e True Ketamine may be indicated in a domiciliary situation but would not be the technique of first choice in hospital.

a True The coeliac plexus innervates the abdominal viscera.
b True But is employed usually for chronic pain relief in association with pancreatic carcinoma.
c False This is possible, but the technique is more likely to be successful when an image intensifier is used. X-ray control is now regarded as mandatory.
d True Due to sympathetic blockade.
e True This is where the coeliac plexus lies.

a True The second division of the trigeminal nerve supplies the nasal area.
b True The third division of the trigeminal nerve supplies this region.
c False The angle of the mandible is supplied by the anterior rami of spinal nerves C2–3.
d False This is supplied by the glossopharyngeal nerve.
e True The auriculotemporal nerve, a branch of the third division of the trigeminal, supplies the tympanic membrane.

a True Nitrous oxide exhibits a depressant effect on methionine synthetase activity after prolonged inhalation.
b True See **a**.
c True See **a**.
d False Although there are megaloblastic changes, these are not attributable to vitamin B_{12} deficiency, nor would this type of anaemia develop in three days.
e False This has not been reported.

30 Helium

a Has a viscosity similar to that of oxygen.

b Is in liquid form in brown cylinders.

c Inhalation causes voice changes.

d Is used to decrease the work of breathing in bronchospasm.

e Supports combustion.

31 The following are appropriate agents for premedication

a Atropine to induce sedation.

b Lorazepam to achieve anxiolysis.

c Hyoscine as an anticholinergic.

d Papaveretum to relieve anxiety.

e Phenothiazines as anticholinergics.

32 Concerning preoperative assessment

a Haemoglobin concentration should be available for all patients undergoing elective surgery.

b A chest X-ray is not required routinely in patients less than 60 years of age.

c A patient with incapacitating disease which constantly threatens life is in ASA grade IV.

d A healthy patient with only mild systemic disease is classed as ASA grade II.

e The mortality rate of patients in ASA grade V approaches 10%.

33 Halothane hepatotoxicity is associated with

a The elderly.

b Obesity.

c Prolonged anaesthesia.

d History of cholecystitis.

e Oxidative enzymatic degradation.

a **True** It may be given accurately at low flows through an oxygen rotameter. Its density is 1/8 that of oxygen. *(Ch. 16, A & S)*

b **False** Helium cylinders contain gaseous helium at room temperature. *(Ch. 17, A & S)*

c **True** Its low density causes a change in the timbre of the voice.

d **False** Helium does not relieve lower airway obstruction. However, it is used commonly as a temporary expedient in upper airway obstruction, when flow is turbulent.

e **False** Helium is non-flammable and does not support combustion.

(Ch. 19, A & S)

a **False** Atropine may cause central stimulation. Hyoscine is more sedative.

b **True** Benzodiazepines possess anxiolytic actions in doses unlikely to produce sedation.

c **True** Hyoscine is an anticholinergic but should be avoided in the elderly because of dysphoria and restlessness.

d **False** Although good sedatives, opioids have poor anxiolytic actions.

e **True** Phenothiazines possess atropine-like actions.

(Ch. 19, A & S)

a **False** Measurement of haemoglobin is necessary for: all patients undergoing major surgery, males over 50 years, all females, and where indicated by the presence of systemic disease.

b **True** But the presence of cardiac or respiratory disease or the likelihood of thoracic surgery indicates the need for this.

c **True**

d **False**

e **True**

(Ch. 9, A & S)

a **False** Hepatoxicity with halothane has been reported in all adult age groups and none predominates.

b **True** Obese patients seem to retain halothane longer than thinner ones, and this seems to predispose to halothane hepatotoxicity.

c **False** A single prolonged anaesthetic is not associated particularly with halothane hepatotoxicity.

d **False** There is no association between cholecystitis and halothane hepatotoxicity.

e **False** The mechanism of hepatotoxicity is associated with reductive enzyme pathways.

34 **Suxamethonium is contraindicated in**

a   Acute intermittent porphyria.

b   Congestive cardiac failure.

c   Chronic renal failure controlled with dialysis.

d   Myotonia dystrophica.

e   A patient who has been paraplegic for one year.

35 **During anaesthesia in a patient with glomerulonephritis for laparotomy**

a   Mannitol 1.5 g/kg should be given.

b   Droperidol should be avoided as it decreases renal blood flow.

c   Halothane should be avoided because it is nephrotoxic.

d   A sympathomimetic should be given to increase glomerular filtration rate (GFR).

e   Alteration in plasma protein concentrations may affect neuromuscular blocking activity.

36 **Postoperative pain may be treated appropriately with**

a   Morphine by infusion to achieve a plasma concentration of 8 ng/ml.

b   I.m. papaveretum in a dose of 20 mg, 4-hourly for a 70 kg adult.

c   Buprenorphine given sublingually.

d   Oral sustained-release preparations of morphine.

e   Bilateral intercostal blocks for upper abdominal surgery.

37 **The management of chronic (intractable) pain in a young adult may include the following.**

a   Frequent i.m. injection of morphine.

b   Oral antidepressants.

c   Intrathecal phenol in glycerine.

d   Facial nerve blockade for unilateral facial pain.

e   Coeliac plexus block for intra-abdominal malignancy.

(Ch. 12, Ch. 41, A & S)

a False Suxamethonium is not contraindicated in acute intermittent porphyria.

b False This is not a contraindication.

c False However, dialysis may lead to a marked reduction in plasma cholinesterase activity.

d True Suxamethonium has been associated with intense muscle rigidity in the presence of myotonia dystrophica.

e False But suxamethonium is contraindicated in early paraplegia because muscular denervation can result in profound hyperkalaemia after its administration.

(Ch. 41, A & S)

a False Mannitol is not indicated in this condition.

b False Droperidol does not decrease renal blood flow.

c False Halothane is not nephrotoxic and is not contraindicated.

d False Sympathomimetic agents cause a reduction in renal blood flow and consequently GFR. *(Ch. 13, A & S)*

e True The albumin: globulin ratio is reversed, and protein binding of neuromuscular agents is altered.

(Ch. 25 A & S)

a False The minimum effective analgesic concentration (MEAC) for morphine infusions is about twice this value (12–24 ng/ml).

b True But conventional i.m. use carries several disadvantages.

c True Buprenorphine is a partial agonist opioid analgesic. However, its use following morphine is not recommended.

d False There is a reduction in the rate of gastric emptying postoperatively, and this may lead to delayed absorption or 'dumping'.

e False Although unilateral blockade is recommended after cholecystectomy through a subcostal incision, bilateral block is not recommended because of the risk of pneumothorax.

(Ch. 43, A & S)

a False Injections should be avoided for long-term therapy. Oral or rectal administration is preferred.

b True Analgesic activity of opioids may be enhanced by concurrent administration of a tricyclic antidepressant.

c True Dermatomal analgesia can be achieved with correct positioning of the patient during intrathecal injection.

d False The facial nerve is motor to the facial muscles. Trigeminal nerve blockade may be appropriate treatment of facial pain.

e True Pain arising as a result of pancreatic neoplasia responds to injection of alcohol to the coeliac plexus.

38   Hazards in the operating theatre are minimised if

a   A theatre temperature of 22–24°C is combined with a relative humidity of 50%.

b   Cyclopropane is used in oxygen only.

c   Volatile agent concentration in the atmosphere is limited to 25 parts per million (ppm) by the use of scavenging apparatus.

d   Needles are never resheathed when a patient with hepatitis B is undergoing anaesthesia.

e   Re-usable equipment is soaked in 2% glutaraldehyde for 3 hours following use on a patient with AIDS.

39   Cardiac arrhythmias during halothane anaesthesia.

a   Are less frequent during light anaesthesia.

b   Are more frequent during hypercapnia.

c   Can be terminated using a beta-blocker.

d   Are more frequent in the presence of hyperkalaemia.

e   May result in a reduction of blood pressure.

40   Nitrous oxide

a   Decreases the ventilatory response to hypercapnia.

b   Is slightly less soluble than nitrogen in blood.

c   May be associated with postoperative hearing loss.

d   May be associated with bone marrow dysplasia after prolonged administration.

e   Does not support combustion.

41   The pressure in a half-filled nitrous oxide cylinder depends upon

a   The percentage of liquid N_2O present.

b   The ambient temperature.

c   The saturated vapour pressue of N_2O.

d   The molecular weight of N_2O.

e   The pseudo-critical temperature.

(Ch. 18, A & S)

a True Patients are at risk of hypothermia at an ambient temperature below 21°C. Neonatal surgery demands higher ambient temperatures. *(Ch. 34, A & S)*

b False Cyclopropane is explosive in oxygen (2–60%) as well as in air.

c False The recommended maximum concentration of volatile agents in the theatre environment is 2 ppm. However, hazards to theatre staff as a result of occupational exposure to pollutants may have been exaggerated.

d True Resheathing of needles is not recommended.

e True Thorough washing before immersion is recommended. Disposable equipment should be used whenever possible.

(Ch. 9, A & S)

a False They are more frequent during light anaesthesia.

b True Hypercapnia provokes sympathoadrenal activity.

c True But beta-blockers must be used with caution in the presence of halothane; excessive doses may cause bradycardia and profound hypotension.

d True Ventricular arrhythmias arise with hyperkalaemia.

e True But usually there is little effect.

(Ch. 9, A & S)

a True There is mild depression of the ventilatory response to carbon dioxide.

b False The blood gas solubility coefficient of nitrous oxide is 0.47, and of nitrogen 0.015. *(Appx. II, A & S)*

c True Caused by diffusion into the middle ear with a consequent increase in pressure.

d True This results from suppression of vitamin B_{12} and methionine synthetase activity. This can occur after short anaesthesia in critically ill patients.

e False Nitrous oxide supports combustion, although it is not flammable.

(Ch. 17, A & S)

a False This does not influence the pressure in the cylinder.

b True Temperature influences the saturated vapour pressure.

c True It is the only property of the agent which determines pressure in the cylinder. *(Ch. 16, A & S)*

d False

e False This relates to Entonox. It is the temperature at which Entonox separates into its constituent parts . *(Ch. 33, A & S)*

42   The Mapleson A breathing system

a   Is a partial rebreathing system.

b   Requires a fresh gas flow (FGF) rate of 2 × minute volume to prevent rebreathing of alveolar gas during spontaneous ventilation.

c   Requires a fresh gas flow rate of 3 × minute volume to prevent rebreathing of alveolar gas during spontaneous ventilation.

d   Requires 100 ml/kg fresh gas flow during IPPV.

e   Forms the basis of the Lack system.

43   Control of intraocular pressure during induction of anaesthesia

a   Concerns the same factors as those controlling intracranial pressure.

b   Can be achieved safely with ketamine.

c   May indicate the need for suxamethonium in the emergency patient with a penetrating eye injury.

d   Is important to minimise loss of vitreous where a penetrating eye injury is present.

e   Is necessary during squint surgery.

44   The Fluotec Mark 3

a   Is a temperature compensated vaporiser.

b   Should be used with a minimum fresh gas flow rate of 3 litre/min.

c   Should be used with a minimum fresh gas flow rate of 2 litre/min.

d   Is affected by back pressure when fresh gas flow rate is greater than 2 litre/min.

e   Can be used as a drawover vaporiser.

45   Postoperative vomiting

a   Is always accompanied by nausea.

b   Is less frequent when hyoscine is given as part of premedication.

c   Increases the risk of postoperative pulmonary atelectasis.

d   Is more likely if opioid analgesics are given postoperatively.

e   Is more common in men than in women.

a True However, when FGF rate = alveolar minute ventilation, only dead space gas is re-breathed.

b False See **a**. *(Appx. VII, A & S)*

c False See **a**.

d False Usually at least 2.5–3 times the minute volume is required.

e True The Lack is a coaxial form of the Mapleson A.

a True Pa_{CO_2} is a major determinant of IOP. Other factors include Pa_{O_2}, posture and venous drainage.

b False Ketamine increases IOP.

c True Suxamethonium is indicated during rapid sequence induction when difficulty is anticipated with tracheal intubation in an unfasted patient.

d True Vitreous prolapse may occur with acute increases in IOP.

e False Extraocular surgery may be performed under any suitable anaesthetic technique.

a True The mechanism is a bimetallic strip.

b False The Mark 3 is accurate down to a fresh gas flow rate of less than 1 litre/min.

c False See **b**.

d False The Mark 3 Fluotec is unaffected by back pressure.

e False The internal resistance is too high to be used in this way.

a False Vomiting is not invariably associated with nausea.

b True Hyoscine possesses anticholinergic actions which confer an anti-emetic action.

c True Secondary to the risk of aspiration.

d True Opioid analgesics have an emetic action.

e False It tends to be more common in women.

46 **The following breathing systems require a fresh gas flow rate greater than the patient's minute volume to prevent rebreathing of carbon dioxide during spontaneous ventilation**

a Magill.
b Mapleson E.
c Lack.
d Circle system with CO_2 absorption.
e Mapleson C.

47 **A Wright respirometer may be used alone to measure**

a Tidal volume.
b Peak flow rate.

c Anatomical dead space.

d Minute volume.
e Functional residual capacity (FRC).

48 **Central cyanosis in a patient in the immediate postanaesthetic recovery period may be due to**

a Shivering.

b Replacement of blood by crystalloid fluid.

c Malignant hyperthermia.
d Diffusion hypoxia.

e Low cardiac output.

49 **The following occur frequently in the early postoperative period**

a Hypertension.

b Hypocalcaemia.

c Decreased lipolysis.

d Shivering.
e Suxamethonium pains.

a **False** Fresh gas flow approximating to the alveolar minute volume ensures efficient carbon dioxide elimination.
b **True** 2.5–3 × minute volume is required.
c **False** The Lack system is a coaxial form of the Magill (Mapleson A) system.
d **False** A fresh gas flow rate of less than 1 litre/min may be used.
e **True** It is an inefficient breathing system and requires a fresh gas flow rate of 2.5 × minute volume.

a **True** But it is inaccurate at very high or very low tidal volumes.
b **False** Used in this way damage may result to the vanes of the respirometer.
c **False** Measurement of carbon dioxide concentration is required as well as volume.
d **False** A stopwatch will be required!
e **False** FRC is measured by the helium dilution method.

a **True** Shivering increases oxygen demand. Desaturation of arterial blood may result unless supplemental oxygen is supplied.
b **False** With haemodilution, insufficient desaturated haemoglobin may be present for cyanosis to be detected.
c **True** Malignant hyperthermia may arise in the postoperative period.
d **True** Oxygen should be given in the immediate postoperative period to all patients who have been breathing a nitrous oxide/oxygen mixture.
e **True** Because of resultant increased venous admixture.

a **True** This may occur as a manifestation of pain, hypoxaemia, hypercapnia, etc.
b **False** But reduction in ionised calcium (Ca^{++}) may occur transiently with hyperventilation.
c **False** The catabolic response to surgery results usually in increased lipolysis.
d **True** Commonly after volatile agents. Oxygen should be administered.
e **False** The incidence is 50% in those receiving the drug, but the onset is usually related to ambulation.

50   Heat loss during surgery can be minimised by

F   a   Maintaining environmental temperature at 20°C.

T   b   The use of a heat-reflecting blanket intraoperatively.

F   c   Administration of i.v. fluids via central lines.
T   d   Humidification of inspired gases.

F   e   Small doses of phenothiazines.

51   Ketamine hallucinations are less troublesome

T   a   In children.
T   b   With diazepam premedication.

F   c   With an opioid premedication.
F   d   In outpatients.

T   e   By recovery in quiet surroundings.

52   Waste gas scavenging systems

F   a   Present significantly increased resistance to expiration.

F   b   May employ activated charcoal.
F   c   Should incorporate an active disposal system.

F   d   Employ connectors of 19 mm diameter to avoid cross connections.

T   e   Employ negative pressure valves in the system.

(Ch. 23, A & S)

a False The thermoneutral environmental temperature for an unclothed adult is 27°C. Theatre temperature is usually maintained at about 22°C.

b True Covering exposed surfaces with heat-reflecting foil minimises heat loss.

c False Warming of i.v. fluids is recommended to minimise heat loss.

d True Inhalation of cold dry gases necessitates heating and humidification by the respiratory tract. Humidification of inspired gases reduces loss of latent heat of vaporisation.

e False Small doses of phenothiazines act as vasodilators and reduce core temperature.

(Ch. 10, A & S)

a False But children may not report hallucinations.

b True Diazepam and lorazepam have been advocated as premedicants to reduce the emergence phenomena associated with ketamine.

c False Opioids may cause dysphoric reactions.

d False Ketamine is generally considered to be an unsuitable agent for outpatient anaesthesia.

e True It is recommended that patients who have received ketamine should be nursed in quiet surroundings consistent with normal observation of airway and vital signs.

(Ch. 17, A & S)

a False Resistance to expiration is not normally increased. Care should be exercised in positioning tubing to avoid accidental compression.

b True Activated charcoal may be employed to adsorb volatile agents.

c False Passive and active systems are available. An active system is not always necessary.

d False Connectors are of 30 mm diameter to avoid inadvertent connection to anaesthetic delivery systems.

e True Negative pressure relief valves prevent transmission of negative pressure to the system.

[handwritten: Can use ketamine for TIVA]

53 Concerning total i.v. anaesthesia

a Ketamine can be employed. *[handwritten: F / T]*

b Can be employed safely in the presence of upper airway obstruction. *[handwritten: F]*

c Requires a loading dose at induction. *[handwritten: T]*

d Depth of anaesthesia is judged by eye signs. *[handwritten: F]*

e Nitrous oxide/oxygen cannot be used in conjuction. *[handwritten: T]*

54 Inguinal herniorrhaphy can be performed under the following types of anaesthesia:

a Paravertebral block at T10–12. *[handwritten: F < T, L, L2, 10 mg/ml]*

b Epidural block using 20 ml lignocaine 1% at L3–4. *[handwritten: T, = 200 mg]*

c Saddle block. *[handwritten: F]*

d Caudal block with 3 ml 0.5% cinchocaine. *[handwritten: F]*

e Subarachnoid block using 3 ml of heavy bupivacaine 0.5%. *[handwritten: T]*

55 Hypertension in the postoperative period is commonly due to

a Hypocapnia. *[handwritten: F]*

b Phaeochromocytoma. *[handwritten: F]*

c Full bladder. *[handwritten: T]*

d Surgical pain. *[handwritten: T]*

e Volatile anaesthetic agents. *[handwritten: F]*

[handwritten margin notes: ↓CO₂   ↑CO₂ ... causes ...]

[handwritten bottom notes:
Prilocaine   7
bupivacaine   2
lignocaine   5 / 7
mg/kg]

a True   Ketamine can be used as the sole anaesthetic agent but its use must be preceded by the injection of atropine. *(Ch. 10, A & S)*

b False   Airway patency *must* be ensured before the use of any intravenous anaesthetic agent.

c True   In order rapidly to achieve the steady state condition at which infusion rate is equal to elimination rate, a loading dose is given. *(Ch. 8, A & S)*

d False   Eye signs originally described by Guedel are not a reliable monitor of non-inhalational anaesthesia. *(Ch. 20, A & S)*

e True   If nitrous oxide is used, the technique cannot be total intravenous anaesthesia.

(Ch. 26, A & S)

a False   Injection should be performed at T11, T12, L1 and L2.

b True   This is an acceptable technique for inguinal herniorrhaphy.

c False   A saddle block affects only the lower sacral segments, which form a ring around the anus. This is an unsuitable block for herniorrhaphy.

d False   Cinchocaine is no longer available. Three millilitres of local anaesthetic injected into the caudal space produces minimal spread of anaesthesia.

e True   This should produce an adequate block for inguinal herniorrhaphy.

(Ch. 24, A & S)

a False   Hypocapnia alone does not produce hypertension.

b False   Phaeochromocytoma is a very rare cause of hypertension in the postoperative period.

c True   A full bladder can be very distressing and can result in an increase in arterial pressure.

d True   Surgical pain may have either a hyper- or a hypotensive effect and should be corrected before other causes of deranged arterial pressure are investigated.

e False   All volatile anaesthetic agents depress the cardiovascular system and do not cause hypertension in the postoperative period.

56   A young healthy adult presents for thyroidectomy

a   Preoperative thyroid function testing is indicated.

b   Thoracic inlet X-rays are indicated preoperatively.

c   Preoperative beta-blockers may be indicated.

d   Lugol's iodine should be given preoperatively to reduce vascularity.

e   Postoperative respiratory obstruction may occur due to tracheal collapse.

57   The following techniques are appropriate during reduction of dislocation of the shoulder

a   Bier's block.

b   Axillary brachial plexus block.

c   Interscalene block.

d   General anaesthesia.

e   Diazepam sedation.

58   Static electricity

a   Can cause a hypoxic mixture to be given via the rotameters.

b   Is produced by two non-conducting surfaces.

c   Is removed by wetting the surfaces.

d   Is reduced by ionising radiation.

e   Is reduced by the use of a conducting breathing system.

(Ch. 41, A & S)

a **True** Hyperthyroidism must be corrected before elective surgery.
b **False** If the possibility of retrosternal spread of tumour is present or if tracheal compression is suspected, neck and thoracic inlet X-rays should be requested.
c **True** Control of symptoms may be achieved by preoperative oral treatment with beta-blockers. Treatment should continue into the postoperative period.
d **False** Potassium iodide t.i.d. has superseded the use of Lugol's iodine solution.
e **True** Pressure exerted by a goitre may erode the tracheal cartilage and result in loss of support. Such patients present with airway obstruction on inspiration. *(Ch. 24, A & S)*

(Ch. 26, A & S)

a **False** A Bier's block (IVRA) does not anaesthetise the shoulder as the tourniquet is placed on the upper arm!
b **False** This would anaesthetise the lower arm well, but not the shoulder.
c **True** A brachial plexus block, using the interscalene approach, could be used to reduce a dislocated shoulder but is not performed commonly in this situation.
d **True** General anaesthesia can be used.
e **False** Diazepam is required in anaesthetic doses for reduction of a dislocated shoulder, and other techniques are more appropriate.

(Ch. 16, Ch. 17, A & S)

a **True** Modern rotameters incorporate antistatic devices, but static electricity can cause the bobbins to stick to the side of the tube and provide a false indication of flow.
b **True** It is necessary for two non-conducting surfaces to allow the build-up of charge.
c **True** Wetting the surface decreases insulation and increases conductivity.
d **False** The static charge on a surface may be increased by ionising radiation due to displacement of electrons.
e **True** Although flammable anaesthetic agents are rarely used, the presence of the yellow stripe on black rubber indicates conductivity of the breathing system, and this minimises the build-up of static charge.

59   Inhalational induction may be used in the following circumstances

a   Acute epiglottitis.

b   A patient with a 'full stomach'.

c   Bronchopleural fistula.

d   Tension pneumothorax.

e   Maxillary fracture.

60   Nasotracheal intubation is contraindicated in the following

a   Fractured base of skull.

b   Exodontia.

c   A patient with a bleeding diathesis.

d   Guillain-Barré syndrome.

e   Uncomplicated myocardial infarction.

61   The following structures are traversed during midline lumbar epidural puncture

a   Ligamentum flavum.

b   Supraspinous ligament.

c   Ligamentum denticulum.

d   Posterior longitudinal ligament.

e   Stratum spinosum.

a True This is the method of choice. Intravenous injection before anaesthesia may precipitate complete airway obstruction. *(Ch. 34, A & S)*

b False Rapid sequence intravenous induction is mandatory in such cases. *(Ch. 32, A & S)*

c True It is necessary to avoid contamination of the 'good' lung and avoid producing a pneumothorax with IPPV. Inhalational induction in the sitting position is a useful option before insertion of a double-lumen tube. *(Ch. 39, A & S)*

d False Anaesthesia should not be given in the presence of a tension pneumothorax. Nitrous oxide increases the pressure in a pneumothorax. An underwater seal drain is mandatory before anaesthesia. *(Ch. 23, A & S)*

e False The potential for bleeding in the upper airway precludes the use of inhalational induction. Rapid sequence induction with suction apparatus immediately to hand is the method of choice.

---

a True Nasal haemorrhage may result and the potential for introduction of infection exists.

b False A nasal tube permits access to the mouth during dental surgery and allows better positioning of a throat pack. *(Ch. 35, A & S)*

c True Haemorrhage following trauma to the nasopharyngeal mucosa is a complication of nasal intubation. *(Ch. 20, A & S)*

d False Long-term tracheal intubation may be required and the nasal route carries some advantages in this respect. *(Ch. 20, Ch. 41, A & S)*

e False When tracheal intubation is required, there is no contraindication to the use of the nasal route.

---

a True The epidural needle passes in turn through the supraspinous ligament, interspinous ligament and the ligamentum flavum.

b True See a

c False The ligamentum denticulum lies within the subarachnoid space and is attached to the spinal cord.

d False The posterior longitudinal ligament is not traversed during lumbar epidural puncture.

e True This is part of the epidermis of the skin which is traversed during epidural puncture.

62 **The following disinfectants are effective decontaminants in a breathing system**

a Ethylene oxide.

b Chlorhexidine hydrochloride in spirit.

c Chlorhexidine hydrochloride in water.

d Glutaraldehyde for 3 hours.

e Cetrimide solution BPC (1%).

63 **The following are common causes of hypotension during anaesthesia**

a Hypercapnia.

b Hypovolaemia.

c Vecuronium.

d Gallamine.

e Isoflurane.

64 **Nitrous oxide**

a Is taken up rapidly and anaesthesia is rapidly attained.

b Cylinders contain small amounts of nitric oxide and nitrogen dioxide.

c Can give rise to bone marrow depression.

d Can give rise to methaemoglobinaemia after prolonged administration.

e Lowers the MAC of a concurrently administered agent.

65 **When administering anaesthesia to a patient suspected of being susceptible to malignant hyperpyrexia (MHS)**

a Premedication with morphine and atropine is acceptable.

b Pancuronium is a good choice of muscle relaxant.

c Nitrous oxide should be avoided.

d Dantrolene should be immediately available.

e Regional blockade is a safe technique.

a True The gas may be explosive in air and is commonly used in combination with carbon dioxide.
b False Chlorhexidene in alcohol is used as a skin preparation preoperatively.
c False Aqueous chlorhexidine may be used for bladder irrigation and catheter lubrication.
d True After prior washing in soap and water.
e False Cetrimide, which also has detergent properties, is used predominantly for skin disinfection. *(Ch. 13, BNF)*

---

a False Hypercapnia leads to myocardial stimulation and hypertension.
b True Hypovolaemia due to either preoperative fluid loss or surgical blood loss results in hypotension.
c False Vecuronium has no actions on the cardiovascular system. *(Ch. 12, A & S)*
d False Gallamine causes a tachycardia and its use is unlikely to result in hypotension. *(Ch. 12, A & S)*
e True Isoflurane causes peripheral vasodilatation and hypotension with a reactive tachycardia. *(Ch. 9, A & S)*

---

a True The low blood/gas partition coefficient of nitrous oxide (0.45) allows rapid equilibration between inspired and alveolar concentrations.
b False These contaminants of the production of nitrous oxide are removed by scrubbing at the manufacturing stage. Serious complications may result if these contaminants remain.
c True This is due to methionine synthetase depression.
d False This is not a feature of nitrous oxide usage.

e True The MAC of an agent is determined with reference to its administration in oxygen alone, and remains constant with concurrently administered agents. However, MAC values are additive.

---

a False Anticholinergic agents are contraindicated in an MHS patient.
b True Pancuronium is deemed to be free of triggering potential.
c False Nitrous oxide may be employed in the MHS patient.
d True This is the specific treatment for MH and may be administered preoperatively as prophylaxis in the MHS patient.
e False MH has occurred in association with spinal blockade.

Pipeline pressure = 400 kPa

66   Severe pulmonary barotrauma may be avoided by

a   A compliant reservoir bag.

b   Supplying gas by pipeline rather than by cylinder.

c   Use of non-interchangeable breathing system connections.

d   Use of a blow off valve at 33 kPa in the inspiratory limb.

e   A blow off valve of 7 kPa on the machine.

reservoir bag → limits P in bsyst to 30mmH2O = 3kPa

blow off valve 33kPa 330mH — 7s wreo machi

67   The following would be noticed within 10 minutes of intubation of the right main bronchus

a   High ventilation pressure.
b   Increased requirement for anaesthetic vapour.   *induchai*

c   Collapse of right upper lobe.

d   Hypercapnia.

e   Hypotension.

68   Ruptured pulmonary alveolus may cause

a   Subcutaneous emphysema.

b   Pneumopericardium.

c   Superior vena cava syndrome.

d   Pneumomediastinum.
e   Tension pneumothorax.

(Ch. 17, A & S)

a True A compliant reservoir bag in the breathing circuit limits the pressure in the breathing system to approximately 30 cmH$_2$O (3 kPa).

b False The pipeline pressure of 400 kPa is capable of causing severe pulmonary barotrauma.

c False Breathing system leaks under conditions of high pressure are more likely with interchangeable connections.

d False A blow-off valve at 33 kPa (which is usually incorporated in the anaesthetic machine) protects only the machine components, not the patient.

e True Limiting the circuit pressure to 70 cmH$_2$O (7 kPa) with a blow-off valve obviates serious barotrauma in most patients, although it may still occur in neonates, infants and patients with some pulmonary diseases (e.g. lung bullae).

(Ch. 23, A & S)

a True Tidal volume for two lungs is delivered to one lung only.

b True During the induction phase, shunting of blood through the non-ventilated lung results in a decreased arterial anaesthetic concentration. *(Ch. 8, A & S)*

c False The cuff may occlude the right upper lobe bronchus, but if so, collapse supervenes at a later time.

d False Carbon dioxide elimination remains unchanged. Alveolar ventilation is increased slightly because dead space is reduced, but CO$_2$ elimination is impaired slightly by increased shunt and the net effect is no change during spontaneous or mechanical ventilation.

e False Hypotension would not be expected.

(Ch. 8, D)

a True If a large amount of air escapes rapidly into the mediastinum it may track into the soft tissues of the neck to produce subcutaneous emphysema.

b False The pericardial sac is isolated from any mediastinal air emanating from a ruptured alveolus.

c False The superior vena cava syndrome results from distension of the veins draining into the superior vena cava. It is associated usually with advanced carcinoma of the lungs and can be very unpleasant. It is not usually associated with pulmonary alveolar rupture.

d True Air escaping from ruptured alveoli may track into the mediastinum.

e True Tension pneumothorax is not common with a ruptured alveolus but is possible. The risk is increased in the presence of positive pressure ventilation. *(Ch. 23, A & S)*

69   Regurgitation of gastric contents is likely

a   In a patient with a hiatus hernia.

b   When the lower oesophageal barrier pressure is increased.

c   In the presence of anticholinergic drugs. → reduce LOSP

d   If the patient has not eaten solid food for 4 hours.
    anticholinergic

e   In a patient following minor trauma.

70   Epidural anaesthesia

a   May be performed at any vertebral level. → T

b   Expands the capacity of the intravascular compartment.

c   Eliminates the risk of vomiting and regurgitation.

d   Is associated with urinary retention.

e   Bupivacaine 0.75% is a suitable agent. × T but not for obs

71   After suxamethonium 50 mg, apnoea persists after one hour

a   Probably an atypical cholinesterase is present.

b   Treatment with stored blood is indicated.

c   Treatment with cholinesterases is indicated.

d   This may be due to low serum K+ concentration.

e   Screening of the patient's family is mandatory.

72   In a patient with hypokalaemia

a   Muscle weakness is present.

b   The ECG shows tall T waves.

c   Alkalosis exacerbates the hypokalaemia.

d   The maximum rate of replacement should not exceed 0.5
    mmol/kg/per hour.

e   Digoxin therapy should be withdrawn.

(Ch. 32, A & S)

a True Loss of the anatomical sphincter action of the diaphragm increases the likelihood of regurgitation. Antacid prophylaxis is required for elective as well as emergency surgery.

b False Increased lower oesophageal sphincter (LOS) barrier pressure reduces the risk of reflux of gastric contents into the oesophagus.

c True Anticholinergic drugs reduce LOS pressure.

d True Under normal circumstances, gastric emptying removes solid food only after 6 hours. However, trauma occurring soon after a meal may inhibit gastric emptying for a considerable time.

e True Particularly when trauma occurs soon after a meal.

(Ch. 26, A & S)

a True However, it is performed usually in the thoracic, lumbar or caudal regions.

b True This is due to sympathetic blockade.

c False Vomiting and regurgitation are possible during epidural anaesthesia for surgery, and appropriate precautions, such as starvation and the use of antacids, should be taken.

d True The lack of sensory and motor function can lead to urinary retention.

e True Bupivacaine 0.75% is a suitable agent for epidural anaesthesia, but its use is not approved for obstetric procedures.

(Ch. 12, A & S)

a True A normal dose of suxamethonium produces prolonged paralysis in patients with atypical cholinesterase.

b False Stored blood does not contain normal plasma cholinesterase enzyme activity.

c False No such preparation exists.

d False Hypokalaemia exerts no effect upon depolarising block. In contrast, hypokalaemia may hinder reversibility of nondepolarising muscle relaxants.

e False However, it is advisable to investigate the patient's family as well as the patient for abnormal cholinesterase variants.

(Ch. 22, A & S)

a True Muscle weakness and paralytic ileus may occur when total body potassium is depleted.

b False Tall T waves are characteristic of hyperkalaemia.

c True Alkalosis causes shift of extracellular potassium to the intracellular compartment and exacerbates hypokalaemia.

d True This permits equilibration with the intracellular compartment.

e False But hypokalaemia increases the risk of digoxin toxicity and calls for careful monitoring.

73 Entrainment ratio of a venturi oxygen mask is affected by

a Back pressure.

b Increase in oxygen flow.

c Size of orifice.

d PIFR.

e Dead space of the mask.

74 Concerning Rotameters on a standard anaesthetic machine in the United Kingdom

a Oxygen is on the right when viewed from the front.

b There is an antistatic coating on the inside of the glass tube.

c They are less accurate if the bobbins are not rotating.

d They employ a variable orifice principle.

e They are not affected by back pressure.

75 Passive scavenging systems

a Require the incorporation of a suction device.

b Can produce a negative pressure under some circumstances.

c Require the use of activated charcoal.

d Produce resistance to expiration of 2 cmH$_2$O at a flow rate of 30 litre/min.

e Are inefficient for scavenging vapours.

76 There is an increased risk of cardiovascular complications associated with elective surgery

a In a patient who has had a myocardial infarction in the previous 6 months.

b When the diastolic arterial pressure exceeds 110 mmHg in an untreated patient.

c In patients over 70 years.

d With mitral stenosis.

e When the 'Goldman score' exceeds 25 points.

(Ch. 16, Ch. 24, A & S)

a True Back pressure reduces air entrainment and increases the delivered concentration of oxygen.

b False The entrainment ratio remains constant over a range of gas flows.

c True The various oxygen concentrations required are attained by using orifices of different diameter.

d False The PIFR does not affect the entrainment ratio. However, the total gas flow into the mask must exceed PIFR to avoid dilution of the oxygen/air mixture by air entrained through the vents in the mask.

e False High dead space may increase the risk of rebreathing alveolar gas when variable performance devices are employed.

(Ch. 16, Ch. 17, A & S)

a False In the flowmeter bank, oxygen is conventionally on the extreme left. However, for reasons of safety, the oxygen is added downstream from the other gases in modern anaesthetic machines.

b True This is to prevent sticking of the bobbin flowmeter which would lead to inaccurate flow readings.

c True See above.

d True The glass tube is tapered, and the size of the aperture increases with increasing flow; the weight of the bobbin is matched by the force caused by the pressure difference to maintain flow.

e False Back pressure causes the rotameter to under-read.

(Ch. 17, A & S)

a False The passive scavenging system merely vents expired gases to the outside.

b True Air movement at the outside terminal may create negative pressure. A relief valve at 50 Pa limits this.

c False Activated charcoal is not part of a passive scavenging system. This adsorbs volatile agents.

d False The resistance to gas flow should not exceed 0.5 cmH$_2$0 at 30 litre/min.

e False Gases and volatile agents may be scavenged by such a system.

(Ch. 19, A & S)

a True The risk of perioperative myocardial infarction is approximately 16%.

b True Elective surgery should be deferred in order to instigate treatment.

c True This increases the 'Goldman score'.

d False Aortic valve stenosis but not mitral valve stenosis is associated with an increased risk.

e True Cardiac mortality is greater than 50%.

77   In day case anaesthesia

a   Only patients of ASA grade I are accepted.
b   Anticholinergic premedication is unnecessary.
c   Propofol is a suitable induction agent.

d   Tracheal intubation in children is hazardous.
e   Local anaesthetic nerve blockade is contraindicated because of long lasting paralysis.

78   Oxygen for medical use

a   Is produced by the fractional distillation of air.
b   Has a critical temperature of 36.5°C.
c   Causes bone marrow depression with prolonged exposure.

d   Is supplied in cylinders at a pressure of 137 kPa. 7 bar

e   Dissolves in plasma at a Pa_{O_2} of 13.3 kPa.

79   Complications of supraclavicular brachial plexus block include

a   Pleural puncture.
b   Phrenic nerve block.

c   Intrathecal injection. — interscalene
d   Intra-arterial injection.
e   Ptosis.

80   Fits during or after anaesthesia may be associated with

a   Enflurane.
b   Methohexitone.

c   Ether. — The convulsions v well known

d   Ketamine.

e   Suxamethonium.

a False Patients of ASA grades I and II and, occasionally, III are acceptable.
b True
c True Propofol most nearly meets the criteria of an ideal induction agent for day cases.
d False Provided the correct size of tube is used, this is not hazardous.
e False Local analgesic techniques with or without general anaesthesia are useful for day case surgery.

a True Commercial manufacture involves fractional distillation of liquid air.
b False The critical temperature of oxygen is $-119°C$.
c False Bone marrow depression is attributed to nitrous oxide. Oxygen in prolonged exposure may cause pulmonary toxicity.
d False The pressure in an oxygen cylinder is 13.7 MPa (137 bar; 1987 lb/in^2). (Ch. 17, A & S)
e True At normal arterial tension (13.3 kPa), oxygen dissolves in plasma in a volume of approximately 0.3 ml/100 ml blood.

a True The incidence of pneumothorax is between 0.5% and 6%.
b True For this reason, and the possibility of pneumothorax, bilateral supraclavicular blocks should not be undertaken.
c False This complication is likely only if the interscalene route is used.
d True The subclavian artery lies in the field of injection.
e True This is a manifestation of sympathetic blockade and Horner's syndrome.

a True Particularly with the use of concentrations greater than 3% inspired.
b False Tonic excitatory movements may be associated with the use of methohexitone on induction, but fitting has not been reported.
c True Ether convulsions are a well-known complication of this agent, which is no longer used in the United Kingdom.
d False Ketamine increases intracranial pressure and cerebral metabolic rate, but has not been reported to cause fits.
e False Suxamethonium is a depolarising muscle relaxant which is employed during electroconvulsive therapy to modify the external manifestations of a fit.

81   Characteristics of nondepolarising neuromuscular block include

a   Post-tetanic facilitation.

b   Always prolonged by acidosis. *atracurium Shealdan enhanced in acidosis.*

c   Postoperative muscle pains.

d   Reversible with edrophonium.

e   Development of dual block.

82   The following are true of a Bier's block in a 60-year-old patient

a   30 ml lignocaine 1.5% is an acceptable dose.

b   Prilocaine is not a suitable agent.

c   Systemic toxicity does not occur with an effective tourniquet.

d   The tourniquet can be released safely after 10 minutes.

e   Injection in the antecubital fossa is preferred.

15 mg/ml .

30   600g
15   1g 1.5ml

83   Stages of anaesthesia as described by Guedel

Morphine + atropine

a   Refer to unpremedicated patients.

b   Refer to patients breathing ether.

c   Are divided into four planes.

d   The third stage is divided into four planes.

e   Include measurement of arterial pressure and heart rate.

84   Injection of thiopentone and suxamethonium is followed by muscle stiffness within 15 s. This may be due to

a   Atypical cholinesterase.

b   Myotonia congenita.

c   Familial periodic paralysis.

d   Malignant hyperpyrexia.

e   Dystrophia myotonica.

(Ch. 12, A & S)

a True Post-tetanic potentiation is a characteristic of nondepolarising (competitive) block.

b False Although the action of some nondepolarising muscle relaxants is potentiated by acidosis, the breakdown of atracurium is enhanced in the presence of acidosis.

c False Postoperative myalgia is associated with the use of suxamethonium.

d True Doses of 0.5–1 mg/kg are used for the reversal of neuromuscular blockade.

e False Dual blockade is associated with prolonged use of large doses of depolarising neuromuscular blocking drugs.

(Ch. 26, A & S)

a False 30 ml of lignocaine 1.5% is 450 mg. This exceeds the toxic dose.

b False Prilocaine is the agent of choice for a Bier's block.

c False The leakage of local anaesthetic agent past an effective tourniquet is a well-recognised complication, and systemic toxicity can ensue.

d False It is recommended that the tourniquet be left in place for 20 minutes or longer.

e False High intravascular pressures can be generated, producing leakage beneath the tourniquet.

(Ch. 20, A & S)

a False Premedication with morphine and atropine was used.

b True It was described in patients breathing ether and air.

c False There are four stages. The third stage is divided into four planes.

d True See above.

e False

a False Atypical cholinesterase prolongs the action of suxamethonium. *(Ch. 12, A & S)*

b True Myotonia congenita is one contraindication to administration of suxamethonium. *(Ch. 41, A & S)*

c False Muscle stiffness is not a characteristic of this condition. *(Ch. 23, A & S)*

d False Onset of muscle stiffness would be later than 15 s.

e True This is another contraindication.

85   In outpatient dental anaesthesia

a   Inhalational induction with high (> 80%) concentrations of nitrous oxide is a useful method.

b   A gauze throat pack should be used to obstruct oral breathing.

c   Focal extrasystoles are common.

d   Intravenous induction of anaesthesia may be undertaken with the patient seated in the dental chair.

e   Relative analgesia is useful because the patient need not be accompanied home.

86   During rapid sequence induction of anaesthesia

a   The patient must be on a tipping trolley or table.

b   Suction must be immediately available.

c   100% oxygen is breathed for at least 7 minutes before induction.

d   The cricoid cartilage should be compressed.

e   Thiopentone is given at a rate of 1 ml/3 seconds.

87   The following modify anaesthetic technique for electroconvulsive therapy (ECT)

a   Lithium treatment.

b   Treatment with monoamine oxidase inhibitors (MAOIs).

c   Cerebrovascular accident (CVA) within 3 months.

d   Sensitivity to propofol.

e   The use of unilateral ECT.

88   Entonox

a   Is stored in cylinders at 2000 lb/in².

b   Is approved for use by unsupervised midwives by the Central Midwives Board.

c   Should be stored below −8°C.

d   May depress bone marrow following prolonged administration.

e   Should not be used in the presence of a closed cavity pneumothorax.

a False This outdated technique has no place in modern practice. The F_{IO_2} must be at least 0.3.

b True Correct placement is essential to obstruct oral breathing whilst maintaining a clear nasopharyngeal passage.

c True Arrhythmias occur in approximately 30% of patients and are usually unifocal extrasystoles.

d False Intravenous induction should be undertaken only in the supine patient. There is a risk of hypotension in the seated position.

e True Relative analgesia employs a concentration of approximately 35% N_2O and recovery is rapid. Verbal contact with the patient is maintained throughout.

a True It is essential to be able to initiate a head down tilt and employ pharyngeal suction to assist gravity drainage of any regurgitated gastric contents away from the laryngeal inlet.

b True See above.

c False Preoxygenation should be employed for 3–5 minutes. Four maximal (vital capacity) breaths are an acceptable alternative.

d True Cricoid pressure should be applied by a competent assistant.

e False Rapid sequence induction employs the use of a predetermined dose of induction agent injected rapidly.

a True Lithium potentiates the action of neuromuscular blocking drugs.

b False Opioids (and particularly pethidine) which interact with MAOIs are not used routinely in anaesthesia for ECT.

c True CVA within three months is a contraindication to the use of ECT.

d False Propofol is probably not indicated for induction of anaesthesia for ECT, as there is some evidence that it modifies the convulsion.

e False The technique of anaesthesia for unilateral ECT is no different from that in bilateral ECT.

a True The normal filling pressure of a cylinder is 13.7 MPa (approximately 2000 lb/in²).

b True It is used widely in delivery suites. *(Ch. 33, A & S)*

c False If 'Entonox' is stored below –7°C, it may separate into its constituent parts.

d True The nitrous oxide component of 'Entonox' is responsible for the bone marrow depression following prolonged administration.

e True Nitrous oxide is contraindicated in the presence of air in closed cavities – such as pneumothoraces.

89   Postoperative hypoxaemia may occur as a result of

- F **a**   Mild hypercapnia.
- T **b**   Nitrous oxide diffusion.

- T **c**   Central depression of ventilation.   *vent - pet*

- T **d**   Increased V/Q mismatch.

- F **e**   Fentanyl given 2 hours previously.   *— large doses*

---

90   Bupivacaine   *Marcaine*

- F **a**   Causes depolarisation of nerve membranes.

- T **b**   Is contraindicated for intravenous regional anaesthesia (IVRA).

- T **c**   Has a longer duration of action than lignocaine.
- T **d**   Is metabolised in the liver.   *amide*

- F **e**   Is unsuitable for intrathecal use.

---

91   The neuromuscular blocking drugs in clinical use   *depolarising*

- F **a**   Are all metabolised by acetylcholine.   *nondepoln →*
- F **b**   Exhibit tetanic fade if the block is depolarising.   *tetani c*

- ? **c**   Produce phase II block when curare-like drugs are used.   *non*

- T **d**   Produce post-tetanic facilitation with curare-like drugs.
- T **e**   Produce initial fasciculation when the drug is an agonist.

non depol - tetani c fade
post tetani facilitate

---

92   After massive inhalation of gastric acid the following may result

- T **a**   Lung abscess.

- T **b**   Hypercapnia.

- T **c**   Bacteraemia.

- T **d**   Hypovolaemia.

- T **e**   Destruction of surfactant.

(Ch. 24, A & S)

a False The influence of mild hypercapnia on oxygen transport is minimal.
b False One would not expect diffusion hypoxia to last more than 10 minutes.
c True Due to the persistent action of volatile anaesthetic agents, opioid analgesics, benzodiazepines, barbiturates, etc.
d True Anaesthesia leads to V/Q imbalance which persists into the postoperative period. The effect on Pa_{O_2} is exacerbated by a decrease in cardiac output and hypoventilation.
e True If given in high doses, fentanyl may produce ventilatory depression at this time.

(Ch. 15, A & S)

a False Local anaesthetic agents act by preventing depolarisation of the nerve membranes, probably by blocking the sodium–potassium channels.
b True Bupivacaine is contraindicated for IVRA. Fatalities have been reported following cuff failure.
c True It has a relative duration two to four times that of lignocaine.
d True It is an amide-linked agent and is metabolised by amidases in the liver.
e False It is suitable for intrathecal use in either plain or hyperbaric formulation.

(Ch. 12, A & S)

a False Acetylcholine is the normal transmitter of neuromuscular signals.
b False A tetanic fade is associated with nondepolarising neuromuscular blocking drugs.
c False Phase II block occurs with repeated doses of depolarising agents, not curare-like drugs.
d True This is a characteristic feature of nondepolarising blocking drugs.
e True Fasciculation is a characteristic of depolarising neuromuscular blocking drugs which mimic the action of acetylcholine.

(Ch. 8, D)

a True Lung abscesses may form if death does not precede their development.
b True Severe pulmonary oedema and fibrosis may result in ventilatory failure.
c True Pulmonary complications arise initially from a chemical pneumonitis, but bacteraemia may supervene.
d True Hypovolaemia occurs secondary to extracellular fluid loss into the lung tissue.
e True This leads to the adult respiratory distress syndrome. *(Ch. 42, A & S)*

[handwritten top margin: $\frac{PV}{T}$ $PV = k\theta$]

93 Boyle's Law

F a Relates pressure to temperature.
T b Applies only to ideal gases.
F c Concerns a given mass of gas. → *[handwritten: T relates to fixed mass of gas.]*
T d Relates pressure to volume.
F e Refers to a given volume of gas.

94 Critical pressure is

[handwritten: SVP at critical temp]

F a The pressure above which a liquid cannot evaporate.

F b The pressure above which a cylinder must not be filled.

T c The pressure of vapour in equilibrium with liquid at critical temperature.

F d The pressure below which Entonox must not be stored.

T e Approximately 50 atmospheres for oxygen.

[handwritten: 50 atm -118°C . critical temp + p]

95 Junctional rhythm accompanied by bradycardia

F a Requires immediate treatment and is dangerous.

T — b Occurs commonly during anaesthesia with halothane.
T c Can be produced by hypoxaemia.
F d Can be produced by light anaesthesia.
T e May be responsive to atropine.

[handwritten: hypoxaemia → tachy → Brady]

96 Humidification of inspired gases reduces

T a Drying and crusting of bronchial secretions.
T b Respiratory heat loss.
T c Respiratory water loss.

F d Anatomical dead space.
F e Likelihood of infection.

a False Boyle's Law applies at constant temperature.
b True Gases which are well above their critical temperature behave usually as ideal gases.
c True It relates to a fixed mass of gas.
d True $P \times V = k$ is the annotation for Boyle's Law.
e False It does not refer to a fixed volume of gas.

---

a False The critical pressure is that pressure required to liquefy a gas at its critical temperature.
b False A cylinder is frequently filled with gas to a pressure above its critical pressure – such as an oxygen cylinder.
c True When a liquid is at its critical temperature, it exists in equilibrium as liquid and vapour. The critical pressure is that pressure above the liquid at its critical temperature.
d False Entonox should not be stored below what is termed the 'pseudo-critical temperature'.
e True The critical temperature of oxygen is approximately –119°C, and the critical pressure is approximately 50 atmospheres.

---

a False Provided that the arterial pressure is maintained there is no need for immediate treatment, but close monitoring is essential.
b True Junctional rhythm is common during halothane anaesthesia.
c False Hypoxaemia usually produces tachycardia in the early stages.
d False Light anaesthesia is usually accompanied by tachycardia.
e True Atropine increases the rate of depolarisation of the sino-atrial node because of vagal inhibition.

---

a True Dry crusts may be a problem after prolonged inhalation of dry gases.
b True Heat loss is reduced by humidification.
c True Respiratory water loss necessary to humidify dry gases is reduced when inhaled gases are humidified.
d False Humidification has no effect on dead space.
e False The likelihood of infection may be increased if humidifiers are sterilised inadequately.

97   During external chest compression in CPR

a   The heel of the hand should be over the cardiac apex.

b   The fingers should be in close contact with the chest wall.

c   The elbow should be flexed.

d   Lung inflation should be performed every 15 compressions.

e   Simultaneous chest inflation improves cerebral blood flow.

98   Antagonism of neuromuscular block

a   Can be achieved with edrophonium.

b   Is unnecessary if the train-of-four (TOF) ratio is < 0.3.

c   Occurs only if atropine is used with neostigmine.

d   Is unnecessary if the patient can sustain a head lift for 5 s.

e   Can be achieved with physostigmine.

99   Concerning muscle relaxants

a   Atracurium is broken down by Hofmann degradation.

b   Pancuronium is a steroid.

c   Atracurium causes less histamine release than vecuronium.

d   Alcuronium can be mixed in the syringe with thiopentone.

e   Vecuronium is a pancuronium derivative with minimal cardiovascular properties.

100   Success of cricoid pressure in prevention of regurgitation of gastric contents depends upon

a   Absence of a nasogastric tube.

b   An intact cricoid cartilage.

c   The oesophagus being pressed against the vertebral body.

d   Preoperative administration of H_2-antagonists.

e   Preoxygenation for 5 minutes.

(Ch. 44, A & S)

a False The heel of the hand should be placed on the lower half of the sternum.
b False The fingers should be raised so as not to injure the ribs.
c False The elbows should be locked in extension to reduce fatigue.
d True When the resuscitator is single-handed, two lung inflations should be performed after every 15 chest compressions.
e False Although this may improve aortic blood flow, the simultaneous rise in venous pressure results in impairment of cerebral blood flow.

(Ch. 12, A & S)

a True Edrophonium is a short-acting anticholinesterase.
b False TOF ratio should be greater than 0.7 to achieve adequate neuromuscular transmission.
c False Atropine is used to counteract the unwanted muscarinic actions of anticholinesterases.
d True Sustained head lift is a useful clinical indication of adequate neuromuscular function.
e False Physostigmine is an anticholinesterase with central actions and is unsuitable for reversal of neuromuscular block.

(Ch. 12, A & S)

a True This process is pH and temperature dependent.
b True But it possesses no steroid actions associated with adrenocortical steroids.
c False Atracurium, alcuronium and tubocurarine may release histamine.
d False Precipitation occurs in the syringe and the practice is unsafe.
e True In contrast to pancuronium, vecuronium is not vagolytic and has no sympathomimetic actions.

(Ch. 32, A & S)

a True A nasogastric tube renders the lower oesophageal sphincter incompetent, and may prevent efficient occlusion of the oesophagus behind the cricoid cartilage.
b True In contrast to other tracheal rings, the cricoid cartilage encircles the trachea and permits oesophageal compression.
c True The oesophagus is compressed between the cricoid cartilage and the body of the sixth cervical vertebra.
d False H_2-antagonists increase the pH of gastric contents, but do not influence the risk of regurgitation.
e False This is an important precaution before rapid sequence induction, but does not influence the efficacy of cricoid pressure.

5. Examination 1

---

1   **The following signs may be present in chronic obstructive airways disease (COAD)**

   a   Diminished area of cardiac dullness.

   b   Palpable liver edge.
   c   Finger clubbing.

   d   Cyanosis.

   e   Increased inspiratory rather than expiratory effort.

---

2   **In respect of a cylinder of anaesthetic gas**

   a   The pressure inside a full nitrous oxide cylinder is 120 atmospheres.
   b   The pressure is reduced to a pipeline value of 60 lb/in^2.

   c   The filling ratio of a nitrous oxide cylinder is the ratio of weight of nitrous oxide to the weight of water it would hold.
   d   Cyclopropane cylinders are bright orange in colour.
   e   Entonox should be stored at a temperature above –7°C.

---

3   **Contaminants of nitrous oxide during manufacture include**

   a   Ammonia.

   b   Chlorine.
   c   Nitric oxide.
   d   Nitrogen dioxide.

   e   Nitrogen.

(Ch. 8, D)

a True A diminished area of cardiac dullness is a feature of emphysema which may occur in COAD.

b True Cor pulmonale is a late feature of COAD.

c False Finger clubbing may occur in the presence of carcinoma, chronic intrathoracic suppuration and fibrosing alveolitis and a number of other conditions, but not in COAD.

d True This may occur in severe COAD. There may be associated polycythaemia.

e False Air trapping is a feature of COAD. This occurs in the expiratory phase with increased respiratory effort.

(Ch. 16, Ch. 17, A & S)

a False The pressure is 44 atmospheres (4.4 MPa).

b True This is the pressure which is applied to the needle valves of the Rotameters.

c True The filling ratio is normally about 67%.

d True

e True Separation of liquid nitrous oxide occurs below this temperature, the pseudocritical temperature for Entonox.

(Ch. 9, A & S)

a True Nitrous oxide is produced by heating ammonium nitrate. Ammonia is a potential impurity.

b False There is no chlorine or chloride involved in the reaction.

c True Nitric oxide (NO) is a higher oxide of nitrogen.

d True Nitrogen dioxide (NO_2) is a higher oxide of nitrogen. The higher oxides dissolve in water, form nitrous and nitric acids, and are toxic.

e True

4   In diabetes mellitus

a   Insulin requirements increase during pregnancy.
b   Postural hypotension may occur.
c   Corneal opacities occur.
d   Microvascular complications occur but only in the elderly.

e   Metformin treatment may lead to acidosis.

5   Nitrous oxide

a   Is stored as a liquid.

b   Has a molecular weight of 44.
c   Is manufactured by heating ammonium nitrate.

d   Supports combustion.
e   May contain contaminants which may be detected by starch-iodide paper.

6   Treatment of hypokalaemia is necessary

a   After cardiac bypass surgery.

b   During treatment for diabetic ketoacidosis.

c   After major burns.

d   After depolarising relaxants.

e   During carbenoxolone therapy.

7   In acute appendicitis

a   There is usually obstruction of the appendix lumen.
b   The pain starts typically in the right iliac fossa.
c   The pain is aggravated by movement.
d   Nausea or vomiting is usually present.

e   The white blood cell count may be normal.

(Ch. 12, D)

a True Blood sugar concentration may be labile during pregnancy.

b True This is a result of autonomic neuropathy.

c False There is no increased incidence of cataract in diabetics.

d False Microangiopathy is independent of age (and possibly independent of diabetic control). *(Ch. 12, D)*

e True Lactic acidosis is a recognised complication of treatment with biguanides, of which metformin is the only one available in the UK.

(Ch. 9, A & S)

a True It has a critical temperature of 36.5°C and is stored usually as a liquid at a pressure of approximately 44 bar.

b True

c True The decomposition of ammonium nitrate leads to the formation of nitrous oxide plus water.

d True Whilst not itself flammable, nitrous oxide supports combustion.

e True Starch iodide paper turns blue in the presence of the contaminants of nitrous oxide manufacture.

---

a True This is common after cardiac bypass surgery, and potassium supplementation is usually required. *(Ch. 40, A & S)*

b True Insulin administration activates sodium/potassium exchange in the distal tubule of the kidney, resulting in hypokalaemia. *(Ch. 41, A & S)*

c False Hyperkalaemia would be expected as a result of massive cell destruction. The use of suxamethonium is contraindicated. *(Ch. 6, A & S)*

d False Suxamethonium, the only available depolarising relaxant in the UK, causes mild transient hyperkalaemia.

e True Carbenoxolone has aldosterone-like effects. *(Ch. 9, D)*

(Ch. 9, D)

a True This is caused by swelling of lymphoid tissue in the walls.

b False Initially the pain is central and moves later to the right iliac fossa.

c True Particularly with peritoneal inflammation.

d True But vomiting is less severe than that associated with intestinal obstruction.

e False Fever and toxicity are associated with an elevated white cell count.

8 **The following factors favour a rapid induction with an inhalation agent**

F a High blood/gas partition coefficient.

F b Low alveolar ventilation.

F c Low SVP at 20°C.

F d High concentrations of catecholamines.

T e The second gas effect.

9 **Atrial flutter**

F a Is caused most commonly by ischaemic heart disease.

F b Is identified by 'f' waves at 20/second.

T c Is characterised by a regular arterial pulse.

150/min 60

F d Must not be treated by DC cardioversion.

T e May be prevented by prophylactic administration of digoxin.

10 **Malignant hyperthermia has the following features**

T a Muscle rigidity.

T b Hyperkalaemia.

F c Relaxation following alcuronium.

F d Increased base excess.

T e Family history.

acidotic

11 **The following drugs are halogenated ethers**

T a Isoflurane.

T b Methoxyflurane.

T c Enflurane.

F d Halothane.

F e Trichloroethylene.

a False A low blood/gas partition coefficient (e.g. nitrous oxide) is necessary for rapid induction with an inhalational agent.
b False Increasing alveolar ventilation increases the rate of induction.
c False The saturated vapour pressure at 20°C indicates the maximum concentration of agent that may be administered to a patient. This may limit the use of 'over pressure' to increase the speed of induction.
d False These increase cardiac output and therefore decrease the rate of induction.
e True Rapid uptake of a second gas (nitrous oxide) from the alveoli allows the alveolar concentration of a volatile agent to increase more rapidly in the presence of a high concentration of nitrous oxide, thus favouring rapid induction of anaesthesia. *(Ch. 9, A & D)*

(Ch. 7, D)

a False Mitral valvular disease is the commonest cause in younger patients. In the elderly, there may be no apparent cause or it may occur secondary to hypertension or ischaemic heart disease.
b False The atrial rate is usually about 300/min.
c True There is usually a regular atrioventricular block but the ratio may vary between 2:1 and 4:1.
d False Low energy cardioversion may be effective.
e True

(Ch. 23, A & S)

a True Increased muscle tone may occur following suxamethonium, particularly in young patients.
b True Hyperkalaemia results from cellular breakdown.
c False Muscle relaxants have no effect on muscle itself.
d False Acidosis occurs.
e True Susceptibility to MH is inherited as an autosomal dominant with variable penetrance.

(Ch. 9, A & S)

a True Isoflurane is 1-chloro, 2,2,2-trifluoro-ethyldifluoromethyl ether.
b True Methoxyflurane is 2,2-dichloro, 1,1-difluoroethylmethyl ether.
c True Enflurane is an isomer of isoflurane.
d False Halothane is a halogenated ethane.
e False There is no ether bond in trichloroethylene.

12 The following are true of anaesthesia in a patient on chronic dialysis

a Suxamethonium is contraindicated.

b Halothane may cause dose-related tubular damage.

c Anaesthesia should be postponed if the haemoglobin concentration is <10 g/dl.

d Antihypertensive treatment should be continued preoperatively.

e A sterile laryngoscope should be used.

13 Pulsation in the neck is probably venous if it

a Is diffuse.

b Increases with abdominal pressure.

c Is readily palpable.

d Varies with ventilation.

e Varies with posture.

14 Naloxone may completely antagonise respiratory depression produced by

a Levorphanol.

b Doxapram.

c Pentazocine.

d Nalbuphine.

e Buprenorphine.

15 The following MAC values are correct at normal atmospheric pressure

a Nitrous oxide – 105%.

b Halothane – 1.2%.

c Enflurane – 1.7%.

d Isoflurane – 1.7%.

e Cyclopropane – 1.0%.

a False Provided that serum potassium concentration is normal, there is no contraindication.

b False Halothane is not nephrotoxic.

c False A haemoglobin concentration of less than 10 g/dl is commonly encountered in patients with chronic renal failure.

d True

e False The oropharynx is not sterile.

---

a True This is observed best with the patient reclining at an angle of 45°.

b True This is the hepatojugular reflex.

c False Venous pressure is impalpable.

d True Intrathoracic pressure is transmitted to the intrathoracic veins.

e True When it is very high in cardiac failure, it may be apparent only when the patient stands.

---

a True This is an opioid agonist and its action is antagonised by naloxone. It has a prolonged duration of action (6–10 h), whilst that of naloxone is 15–20 min and therefore a naloxone infusion may be required.

b False Doxapram is an analeptic respiratory stimulant.

c True Naloxone reverses respiratory depression produced by pentazocine which is a μ antagonist and kappa partial agonist. (Ch. 10, A & S)

d True Nalbuphine is a partial agonist at kappa receptors and antagonist at μ receptors. Its actions are antagonised by naloxone which is an antagonist at μ, kappa, and delta receptors.

e False Buprenorphine is a partial agonist at μ receptors and is therefore antagonised theoretically by naloxone. However, buprenorphine has an extremely high receptor affinity, and in standard dosage, naloxone is relatively ineffective.

---

a True

b False Halothane – 0.8%.

c True

d False Isoflurane – 1.2%.

e False Cyclopropane – 9.2%.

16   The pressure gauge on a nitrous oxide cylinder

T   a   May be calibrated in bar.
F   b   Is essential for assessment of the quantity of residual gas in the cylinder.
F   c   Shows a constant pressure as gas runs steadily out of the cylinder at a flow rate of 10 litre/min, provided that the cylinder still contains liquid nitrous oxide.
T   d   May indicate an increase in pressure after the cylinder is turned off after continuous use.
T   e   Measures absolute pressure.

(3)

17   Complications of diabetes mellitus include

T   a   Renal papillary necrosis.
T   b   Abnormal response to a Valsalva manoeuvre.
T   c   Fat atrophy.
F   d   Dupuytren's contracture.
F   e   Chronic pancreatitis.

(3)

18   In comparison with 2.5% thiopentone, 1% methohexitone

F   a   Is more dangerous on intra-arterial injection.
T   b   Is more painful on i.v. injection.
F   c   Causes more cardiovascular depression.
T   d   Causes more abnormal muscle movements.
F   e   Is more irritant when injected into subcutaneous tissues.

(5)

19   Mapleson's classification of anaesthetic breathing systems

F   a   Describes four systems: A B C D.
F   b   Classifies the Bain system as a Mapleson C.
    c   Describes the Magill system as requiring a fresh gas flow rate equal to the minute volume during spontaneous ventilation.
F   d   Describes the T-piece as a Mapleson D.
F   e   Describes the T-piece system as requiring a fresh gas flow rate of 1.5–2 times the patient's minute volume during spontaneous ventilation.

(4)

Magill A.   Bain D.
lach

(Ch. 16, A & S)

a True However, the gauge is frequently calibrated in kPa.
b False Only the weight of the cylinder provides an indication of the amount of residual nitrous oxide.
c False At high flow rates, pressure in the cylinder may decrease because of evaporation of nitrous oxide, and a consequent decrease in temperature and saturated vapour pressure.
d True The cylinder's temperature increases to that of the ambient temperature.
e False The pressure gauge of a cylinder measures gauge pressure (the pressure in excess of atmospheric pressure).

(Ch. 12, D)

a False Glomerulosclerosis is the characteristic renal lesion complicating diabetes mellitus.
b True This is caused by autonomic neuropathy.
c True This may occur at insulin injection sites.
d False This is associated with alcoholic cirrhosis.
e False Approximately 20% of patients with chronic pancreatitis develop diabetes mellitus.

(Ch. 10, A & S)

a False There are fewer sequelae after intra-arterial injection of methohexitone.
b True This is a distinct disadvantage.
c False Hypotension is less profound and of shorter duration than that associated with thiopentone.
d True Movement, coughing and hiccuping occur commonly during induction of anaesthesia with methohexitone.
e False Methohexitone is less irritant.

(Ch. 17, A & S)

a False Systems A to F are described in the Mapleson classification.
b False The Bain system is an example of a Mapleson D.
c False The Magill system functions efficiently during spontaneous ventilation when fresh gas flow rate is equal to the alveolar minute volume.
d False The T-piece is an example of a Mapleson E system.
e False The T-piece requires a fresh gas flow rate of 2.5–3 times the patient's minute volume during spontaneous ventilation.

20   The following statements are true of total intravenous anaesthesia

    a   Ketamine is an appropriate agent.

    b   A loading dose of anaesthetic agent is necessary to achieve smooth anaesthesia.

    c   Cannot be used as part of nitrous oxide/oxygen/relaxant technique.

    d   The patient breathes air/oxygen.

    e   Propofol is a suitable agent in the elderly.

---

21   The following may cause hypokalaemia

    a   Intravenous digoxin.

    b   Addisonian crisis.

    c   Hyperventilation.

    d   Spironolactone therapy.

    e   Respiratory acidosis.

---

22   Hypoalbuminaemia

    a   Is associated with reduction in serum concentration of ionised calcium.

    b   Is a manifestation of hypopituitarism.

    c   May cause tetany.

    d   May be a feature of carcinoma of the oesophagus.

    e   May develop in hepatic cirrhosis.

---

23   Four hours postoperatively, a patient breathing air is distressed, with heart rate of 100 beat/min, BP 170/100 mmHg, Pa_{O_2} 9 kPa, Pa_{CO_2} 7 kPa, HCO_3^- 28 mmol/litre. This is compatible with

    a   Segmental pulmonary collapse.

    b   Septicaemia.

    c   Overtransfusion.

    d   Hypoventilation.

    e   Metabolic acidosis.

(Ch. 10, A & S)

a **True** 'Dissociative' anaesthesia occurs. Premedication with atropine is recommended.

b **True** This is a simple pharmacokinetic principle. *(Ch. 8, A & S)*

c **True** If N_2O/O_2 are used, total i.v. anaesthesia is not provided.

d **True** An increased F_{IO_2} is recommended during general anaesthesia.

e **True** Although a reduced dose rate is advisable.

(Ch. 14, A & S)

a **False** But hypokalaemia potentiates the toxic effects of digoxin.

b **False** Addisonian crisis is associated with hyponatraemia. *(Ch. 12, D)*

c **True** Hyperventilation results in alkalosis and a shift of potassium from extracellular to intracellular fluid.

d **False** Spironolactone is a potassium-sparing diuretic and is an aldosterone antagonist. *(Ch. 14, A & S)*

e **False** The mechanism is the reverse of that associated with hyperventilation.

a **False** The concentration of ionised calcium is increased because of decreased protein binding. *(Ch. 8, A & S)*

b **False**

c **False** Tetany is a manifestation of hypocalcaemia. *(Ch. 12, D)*

d **True** Patients with carcinoma of the oesophagus may be hypoalbuminaemic because of chronic undernutrition, and may benefit from preoperative parenteral feeding. *(Ch. 39, A & S)*

e **True** Because of impaired albumin synthesis by the liver. *(Ch. 10, D)*

(Ch. 24, A & S)

a **False** Carbon dioxide excretion in this condition would be relatively unaffected.

b **False** The arterial pressure and Pa_{CO_2} are incompatible with this diagnosis.

c **False** Hypercapnia is unlikely with overtransfusion, unless the patient develops gross cardiac and respiratory failure.

d **True** The slightly elevated bicarbonate suggests a chronic element.

e **False** In metabolic acidosis, the plasma bicarbonate concentration is decreased. *(Ch. 2, A & S)*

24 **Pulse oximetry**
 a Measures oxygen saturation.

 b Locates the isobestic point of haemoglobin.

 c Functions poorly on negroid skin.
 d Is inaccurate in the presence of carboxyhaemoglobin.
 e Is inaccurate in the presence of fetal haemoglobin.

---

25 **The plasma concentration of a drug which exhibits first order kinetics**
 a Decreases linearly with time after bolus i.v. administration.

 b Plotted against response gives a sigmoid curve.

 c Declines by 50% in proportion to the initial concentration.
 d Increases rapidly during constant i.v. infusion.

 e At steady state with a constant infusion rate, is inversely proportional to the clearance.

---

26 **Pancuronium**
 a Does not cross the placenta in clinically significant amounts.
 b Causes tachycardia.
 c Causes less hypotension than curare.

 d May cause prolonged paralysis in a patient taking streptomycin.

 e Causes dilation of the pupil.

---

27 **Paroxysmal supraventricular tachycardia is**
 a Usually the result of organic heart disease.
 b Associated with the loss of P waves on the ECG.
 c Often terminated by carotid sinus massage.
 d Often terminated by treatment with verapamil.
 e May be associated with polyuria.

(Ch. 21, A & S)

a True Absorption of light measured at two distinct wavelengths permits calculation of saturation.
b False This is the wavelength at which absorption of light is identical for oxygenated and reduced haemoglobin.
c False
d True Carboxyhaemoglobin and methaemoglobin result in inaccuracy.
e False

(Ch. 8, A & S)

a False The plot of drug concentration against time varies with the drug and its metabolic pathways. It is usually an exponential decay.
b False A linear plot of plasma concentration against response gives a hyperbolic curve; plot of the logarithm of concentration against response gives a sigmoid curve.
c False The half-life is inversely proportional to the elimination rate constant.
d False A constant intravenous infusion results eventually in a relatively constant plasma concentration depending on the rate of administration and the rate of excretion of the drug. A bolus intravenous dose gives a rapid increase in plasma concentration.
e True $I = C_{ss} \times Cl$.

(Ch. 12, A & S)

a True Pancuronium crosses the placenta but this is not clinically significant.
b True Pancuronium has significant sympathomimetic activity.
c True Curare may cause marked hypotension because of histamine release and ganglion blockade.
d True The aminoglycoside antibiotics possess neuromuscular blocking properties, and this may potentiate the action of nondepolarising neuromuscular blocking drugs. *(Ch. 19, A & S)*
e False Amongst the nondepolarising drugs, curare has the greatest ganglion-blocking action and it may cause dilation of the pupil, an effect not produced by other drugs in this class.

(Ch. 7, D)

a False But left ventricular failure may accompany the arrhythmia.
b False Atrial depolarisation is normal but accelerated.
c True This simple expedient may be the only treatment required.
d True This may be indicated if the attack is more severe.
e True This may be a feature of prolonged attacks.

28 **The following factors affect flowmeter readings (of the Rotameter type)**

    a   Water condensation inside the tube.

    b   Dirt on the bobbin.

    c   Static electricity.

    d   Gas escaping past the bobbin.

    e   The use of a gas different from that for which the rotameter was calibrated.

29 **Concerning anaesthetic apparatus**

    a   An oxygen failure warning device must operate even in the absence of nitrous oxide.

    b   The Boyle machine can be classed as an intermittent flow device.

    c   With vaporisers in series, the enflurane vaporiser should be closer to the Rotameters than the halothane vaporiser.

    d   When a restriction in the outflow of a Rotameter causes pressure build up, the actual flow is greater than indicated.

    e   The Ruben valve is of the non-rebreathing type.

30 **The following are causes of metabolic acidosis**

    a   Ureterocolic fistula.

    b   Vomiting.

    c   Diarrhoea.

    d CO_2 retention.

    e   Metformin therapy.

31 **In the acute phase following sudden massive haemorrhage there is**

    a   A reduction in CVP.

    b   Widespread vasoconstriction.

    c   An increase in the volume of interstitial fluid.

    d   Decreased secretion of ADH.

    e   Increased plasma concentration of aldosterone.

(Ch. 17, A & S)

a True Water condensing inside the tube causes the bobbin to stick and results in loss of accuracy.
b True Sticking may occur as a result of debris on the bobbin.
c True Static electricity inhibits movement of the bobbin inside the tube and leads to inaccuracy. The inside of the tube is therefore coated with an antistatic film.
d False Gas escaping past the bobbin through the variable orifice is the principle underlying the operation of the flowmeter.
e True Calibration is affected by gas viscosity at low flow rates, and density at high rates. Thus a flowmeter is calibrated specifically for one gas.
(Ch. 16, A & S)

(Ch. 17, A & S)

a True A safe device is that which relies upon a reservoir of compressed oxygen which is filled from the oxygen supply.
b False A continuous flow of gases is supplied by the Boyle machine.
c False The less volatile agent should be placed downstream to avoid contamination of the second agent. Modern machines prevent the use of two agents in series.
d False The Rotameter over-reads.

e True But non-rebreathing valves may not be 100% efficient.

---

a True Caused by colonic absorption of hydrogen ion.
b False Vomiting results usually in metabolic alkalosis.
c True Diarrhoea leads to loss of bicarbonate ions and metabolic acidosis may result. *(Ch. 5, D)*
d False This causes a respiratory acidosis.
e True Metformin is associated with lactic acidosis. *(Ch. 41, A & S)*

(Ch. 32, A & S)

a True The CVP is a good indicator of intravascular volume.
b True Vasoconstriction is part of the sympathetic response to haemorrhage.
c False A shift of interstitial fluid into the intravascular compartment would be expected.
d False There is increased ADH secretion in response to reduction in stretch receptor activity of the atrial volume receptors.
e False Aldosterone is secreted in response to increased plasma concentrations of angiotensin which result from release of renin from the kidney.

32 **The following drugs are peripherally acting adrenergic blockers**

a Propranolol.

b Reserpine.

c Tolazoline.

d Droperidol.

e Methyldopa.

33 **Water intoxication is associated with**

a Confusion.

b Coma.

c Convulsions.

d Increased heart size.

e Hypokalaemia.

34 **A supraclavicular brachial plexus block**

a Can be carried out safely using 30 ml of lignocaine 2% with adrenaline 1:100 000.

b Results in cutaneous anaesthesia in the whole of the upper limb.

c May cause a Horner's syndrome.

d Has a slower onset time than an axillary block.

e Is contraindicated in haemophilia.

35 **The MAC of an agent varies with**

a Age.

b Hypothermia.

c Lipid solubility of the agent.

d Presence of nitrous oxide.

e Premedication.

(Ch. 13, A & S)

a True Propranolol is a peripheral and central acting beta$_1$, and beta$_2$-adrenergic blocking drug.

b False Reserpine acts centrally to cause depletion of neurotransmitters. *(Ch. 2, BNF)*

c True Tolazoline is a peripherally acting alpha-adrenergic blocking drug.

d True The butyrophenones possess mild alpha-adrenergic blocking activity. *(Ch. 11, A & S)*

e False The action of methyldopa – a false transmitter – is almost entirely central.

(Ch. 5, D)

a True This is caused by cerebral oedema, resulting from hyponatraemia.

b True This may result also from cerebral oedema.

c True These may occur in severe water intoxication.

d False

e False Hyponatraemia occurs.

(Ch. 26, A & S)

a False The maximum safe dose of lignocaine (200 mg; 500 mg with adrenaline) is exceeded if lignocaine 2% is used.

b False The intercostobrachial nerve is not included. This carries cutaneous sensation from the upper medial part of the limb.

c True Horner's syndrome is a frequent complication of brachial plexus block.

d False Axillary block is associated with a prolonged time of onset.

e True Regional anaesthetic techniques are contraindicated in the presence of coagulopathies.

(Ch. 9, A & S)

a True The MAC of an agent increases following birth, peaks around the time of puberty and thereafter decreases slowly.

b True The MAC of an agent decreases in the hypothermic patient.

c True There is a linear relationship between oil/gas partition coefficient and MAC.

d True Nitrous oxide reduces MAC, which is determined by reference to the inhalation agent in oxygen alone.

e True Premedication reduces the requirements for an inhalation agent. MAC is determined normally in the unpremedicated state.

36   The following changes support a diagnosis of obstructive jaundice

a   Increased serum acid phosphatase.
b   Increase in red cell fragility.
c   Stercobilinogen deficiency.

d   Increased urobilinogen.

e   Serum aspartate aminotransferase (AST) concentration < 100 IU/litre.

37   A serum sodium concentration of 127 mmol/litre and potassium 6.8 mmol/litre may be found in the following conditions

a   Acute renal failure.
b   Cushing's syndrome.

c   Hypopituitarism.
d   Pyloric stenosis.

e   Renal tubular acidosis.

38   On a modern UK anaesthetic machine

a   The oxygen alarm does not sound if the nitrous oxide is disconnected.
b   The wall gas pipeline supply should be disconnected for the duration of the preoperative check.

c   The TRITEC vaporiser cannot be used when the circle system and CO_2 absorber are in use.

d   When checking for leaks with the common gas outlet blocked, the oxygen flush may be operated.

e   When checking for leaks, the vaporisers should be switched on.

(Ch. 10, D)

a False Serum alkaline phosphatase concentration is increased.
b False
c True Stercobilinogen is decreased and steatorrhea occurs in obstructive jaundice.
d False Urobilinogen is conjugated bilirubin which is reabsorbed via the gut and excreted in the urine; thus its concentration is decreased in obstructive jaundice.
e True Aspartate aminotransferase is liberated following hepatocellular damage but it may increase in severe obstructive jaundice.

---

a True Hyperkalaemia is a feature of renal failure. *(Ch. 4, A & S)*
b False Sodium is retained as a result of increased corticosteroid secretion in Cushing's syndrome. *(Ch. 12, D)*
c True Hypopituitarism is one of the causes of Addison's disease *(Ch. 12, D)*
d False Pyloric stenosis results in alkalosis and hypokalaemia.
(Ch. 34, A & S)
e False In renal tubular acidosis, the underlying defect is diminished sodium/hydrogen ion exchange. Potassium depletion is common in either type 1 (distal) or type 2 (proximal) renal tubular acidosis.
(Ch. 11, D)

(Ch. 17, A & S)

a False The UK standard for oxygen alarms specifies that they are independent of other gas supplies.
b False Where pipelines are supplied to an anaesthetic machine, they should be disconnected only to ascertain the integrity of the supply from the gas outlet to the Rotameter block as in the single hose test.
c False On older anaesthetic machines, an interlock prevented the concurrent use of trichloroethylene and the circle system; on modern machines, this is not so.
d True The oxygen flush emits gas at a pressure of 400 kPa. This pressure applied to the back bar would cause damage to the Rotameter block, and in order to prevent this, a pressure relief valve operating at 35 kPa is inserted downstream of the vaporisers.
e True This reveals failure to mount vaporisers correctly on the back bar, or failure to close filling caps.

39   The volume of one mole of gas

a   Is equal for all ideal gases at standard temperature and pressure (STP).

b   Varies with pressure.

c   Varies with temperature.

d   Is 22.4 litre at room temperature.

e   Is 1 litre at STP.

40   In the event of a failed tracheal intubation in obstetric anaesthesia

a   Cricoid pressure should be maintained.

b   Only three attempts at intubation should be made.

c   Manual lung ventilation should not be attempted.

d   The patient should be allowed to awaken.

e   Isoflurane in oxygen is the safest technique if the operation must proceed.

41   The following anaesthetics may form explosive mixtures when used during the course of a normal anaesthetic

a   Cyclopropane.

b   Halothane.

c   Enflurane.

d   Methoxyflurane.

e   Diethyl ether.

42   The combination of atrial fibrillation and tachycardia may indicate

a   Uncontrolled thyrotoxicosis.

b   Digoxin toxicity.

c   Ventricular bigeminy with escape beats.

d   Hyperkalaemia.

e   Hypokalaemia.

(Ch. 16, A & S)

a True This is an extension of Avogadro's hypothesis.

b True The volume of the gas varies inversely with pressure at constant temperature – Boyle's Law.

c True The volume varies directly with the absolute temperature at constant pressure – Charles' Law.

d False The molar volume of all perfect gases is 22.4 litre at STP.

e False See above.

(Ch. 33, A & S)

a True The risk of regurgitation persists.

b False However, repeated attempts at intubation by the inexperienced may be dangerous.

c False Manual ventilation with 100% oxygen may be necessary.

d True Unless the situation is urgent. Time is required for the anaesthetist to summon help. Regional anaesthesia may also be considered.

e False Spontaneous ventilation using the agent with which the anaesthetist is most familiar is the preferred technique.

(Ch. 9, A & S)

a True Cyclopropane forms an explosive mixture with oxygen and with nitrous oxide throughout the range of anaesthetic concentrations.

b False This is non-flammable and non-explosive at atmospheric pressure.

c False This is non-explosive in clinical concentrations in oxygen or in nitrous oxide.

d False This is non-flammable in ordinary clinical use, but burns at higher concentrations and temperatures.

e True Ether is flammable at concentrations greater than 2%. It is essential to avoid diathermy whilst using ether. *(Appx. II, A & S)*

(Ch. 7, D)

a True This is an important cause of atrial fibrillation, particularly in the elderly.

b False Bradycardia and ventricular ectopic beats are more common with digoxin toxicity.

c False This may be a manifestation of digoxin toxicity.

d False Ventricular fibrillation may occur in the later stages of hyperkalaemia. *(Ch. 5, D)*

e True If this is severe, atrial tachycardia may produce a reduction in cardiac output. *(Ch. 5, D)*

43 **Malignant hyperthermia is treated specifically with**

a Dantrolene.
b Chlorpromazine.
c Sodium EDTA.
d Calcium EDTA.
e Ca^{++}.

44 **Compliance**

a Of the lung alone is greater than the compliance of the lung and chest together.

b Dynamic compliance may be measured only during controlled ventilation.

c Varies directly with age in adults.

d Is greater when supine.

e Increases during prolonged anaesthesia.

45 **The following drug interactions occur**

a Aspirin displaces warfarin from plasma protein binding sites.

b Digoxin is more toxic in the presence of hyperkalaemia.

c Vecuronium precipitates in thiopentone.

d Probenecid enhances the actions of penicillin.

e Morphine delays the absorption of paracetamol.

46 **In the normal ECG**

a There is a Q wave in V_6.
b There is an upright T wave in aVR.

c The S wave is of greater amplitude than the R wave in V_1.

d The PR interval is 0.24 s.

e Depolarisation lasts 200 ms.

(Ch. 23, A & S)

a True This is the only specific treatment for malignant hyperpyrexia.
b False
c False This is used as a chelating agent in the treatment of poisoning.
d False This is used in the treatment of acute poisoning. *(Ch. 17, D)*
e False

(Ch. 2, A & S)

a True The reciprocal of total respiratory compliance is equal to the sum of the reciprocals of each of its constituent parts, that is, lungs and chest wall. Therefore lung compliance must be greater than total compliance.
b False Dynamic compliance may be measured during spontaneous ventilation.
c False There is no relationship between compliance and age in healthy subjects.
d False In the supine position, the weight of the chest wall tends to reduce the value of total compliance.
e False During prolonged anaesthesia, lung compliance tends to decrease but may be restored with a large tidal breath.

a True Aspirin (in common with other NSAID drugs) prolongs the prothrombin time in patients receiving warfarin. *(Appx. 1, BNF)*
b False Hypokalaemia increases the likelihood of toxicity with digoxin. *(Ch. 14, A & S)*
c True This is an important interaction, as precipitation may occur in a cannula injection port when vecuronium follows the injection of thiopentone.
d True Probenecid is excreted by the kidney in preference to penicillin. *(Ch. 10, BNF)*
e True Morphine delays gastric emptying.

(Ch. 7, D)

a True This represents depolarisation of the intraventricular septum.
b False Repolarisation, represented by the T wave, takes place in the opposite direction from that of the major component of the QRS complex.
c True V_1 is a right-sided lead and ventricular depolarisation, represented by the S wave, is directed away from the lead.
d False This represents first degree heart block; the upper limit of normal is 0.2 s.
e True This is much shorter than the duration of depolarisation in skeletal muscle. *(Ch. 3, A & S)*

47   A depolarising block may be produced by

  a   Neostigmine.   *non depol block?*

  b   Suxamethonium.
  c   Atracurium.   *depol block*
  d   Edrophonium.

  e   Gallamine.   *anticholinestase only*

---

48   Pressure   *Pressure -*

  a   Equals force × distance.
  b   Equals force per unit area.
  c   Is the rate of doing work.
  d   Can be measured using a column of mercury.
  e   Is measured in newtons.

                    work = force x distance

**49   The following are true of a supraclavicular approach in comparison
with an axillary approach to brachial plexus block**

  a   There is a greater risk of intravascular injection.
  b   Analgesia of the shoulder is poorer.
  c   It is more likely to fail to block the posterior interosseous nerve.

  d   It is less likely to give analgesia of the forearm.

  e   There is increased incidence of pneumothorax.

---

50   Pain occurs commonly following i.v. injection of

  a   Thiopentone.

  b   Etomidate.

  c   Suxamethonium.

  d   Neostigmine.

  e   Methohexitone.

(Ch. 12, A & S)

a True Although neostigmine is used usually to antagonise neuromuscular block, high doses of neostigmine may lead to a cholinergic block (as in myasthenia gravis) with a depolarising characteristic.

b True

c False This is a nondepolarising (competitive) agent.

d False Theoretically, it should be possible for overdosage with edrophonium to cause a cholinergic block, but its transient action makes this unlikely.

e False This is a nondepolarising agent.

(Ch. 16, A & S)

a False Work is measured as the product of force and distance.

b True *(Appx. I, A & S).*

c False Power is defined as the rate of working.

d True Hence the use of a mercury barometer and a sphygmomanometer.

e False The SI unit of pressure is the pascal (Pa). *(Appx. I, A & S)*

(Ch. 26, A & S)

a False Intravascular injection commonly complicates the axillary approach.

b False Neither approach provides analgesia of the shoulder.

c False This is a branch of the radial nerve and is blocked by both techniques.

d False The axillary approach is more likely to be associated with this problem.

e True The incidence approaches 6%.

(Ch. 10, A & S)

a False Pain may occur with thiopentone, but is rare unless small veins and rapid injection are used.

b True This occurs in up to 80% of patients. It may be reduced by increasing the speed of injection.

c False Suxamethonium is given following induction of anaesthesia, and complaint of pain should not be encountered!

d False Pain on injection is not a feature of the use of neostigmine used either for antagonism of neuromuscular block or for treatment of supraventricular tachycardia.

e True This has an incidence of up to 21%. It may be minimised by the use of a large vein and by analgesic premedication.

51 **Concentrations of the following ions are higher in intracellular fluid than in plasma**

  a Potassium.

  b Sodium.

  c Phosphate.

  d Bicarbonate.

  e Protein.

52 **The following local anaesthetics cause vasoconstriction**

  a Lignocaine.

  b Cocaine.

  c Amethocaine.

  d Procaine. — Vasodilatation

  e Prilocaine.

53 **Successful ulnar nerve block at the elbow results in**

  a Numbness in the dorsal aspect of the little finger.

  b Numbness in the whole of the dorsum of the hand.

  c Paralysis of all the muscles of the thenar eminence.

  d Numbness of the medial aspect of the forearm.

  e Neuroma formation if injection is made into the intercondylar groove.

54 **Physical dependence may be produced by**

  a Phenylbutazone.

  b Pentazocine.

  c Morphine.

  d Buprenorphine.

  e Diazepam.

(Ch. 4, A & S)

a True Potassium is the main cation in the intracellular compartment, with a concentration of approximately 150 mmol/litre.
b False Sodium is the principal extracellular cation.
c True Intracellular phosphates in the form of ATP and AMP comprise messenger systems in the cell. *(Ch. 5, A & S)*
d False Bicarbonate is primarily an extracellular anion which has roles in buffering and CO_2 transport. *(Ch. 2, A & S)*
e False Intracellular protein anions are present in a concentration lower than that in the plasma.

(Ch. 15, A & S)

a False
b True This causes vasoconstriction. It is used for this purpose in ENT surgery.
c False This has no vasoconstrictor properties. It is used for topical anaesthesia in ophthalmology.
d False This causes vasodilatation; for this reason adrenaline is generally added to solutions of procaine.
e False

(Ch. 26, A & S)

a True The sensory distribution of the ulnar nerve is to the medial one-and-a-half fingers.
b False See above
c False Ulnar nerve block results in paralysis of the hypothenar muscles and adductor pollicis.
d False The median aspect of the forearm is supplied by the medial cutaneous nerve of the forearm which arises from the brachial plexus.
e True Compression of the nerve may be produced by injection of local anaesthetic at this site. It is advisable to inject at a point approximately 2–3 cm proximal to the medial epicondyle.

---

a False
b True Pentazocine is an opioid analgesic with agonist/antagonist properties and physical dependence is well recognised with this agent; it is now a controlled drug – Schedule 3, Misuse of Drugs Regulations 1985. *(Ch. 4, BNF)*
c True Morphine also is a controlled (Schedule 2) drug.
d True Buprenorphine is a controlled (Schedule 3) drug which is subject to safe custody regulations. *(Ch. 11, A & S)*
e True Physical dependence has been reported with the benzodiazepines. *(Ch. 4, BNF)*

55 **The burned patient**

T **a** May develop a high blood concentration of carbon monoxide.

F **b** Hypoventilates in the early phase of injury.
F **c** Requires i.v. fluid therapy when the burn area is > 15%.
F **d** Requires i.v. fluid replacement given totally as albumin solution.
F **e** Should not receive suxamethonium in the acute phase.

after 24hrs → 6olls

---

56 **Hexamethonium**

  a Is a competitive antagonist.

  b Is a parasympathetic ganglion blocker.
  c Does not lead to cycloplegia.
  d Causes depression of respiration.
  e Is excreted by the renal tubule.

---

57 **The critical temperature of a gas is the temperature**

  a At which latent heat of vaporisation is zero.

F **b** At which latent heat of vaporisation is maximum.
F **c** Where it solidifies.
  d Where it liquefies when critical pressure is applied.

T **e** Above which the gas cannot liquefy however high the pressure.

---

58 **Atrial tachycardia with atrioventricular block**

F **a** Has a ventricular rate of 140–220 beat/minute.
F **b** May be caused by digoxin overdose.
T **c** May be converted to sinus rhythm by intravenous propranolol.
T **d** Is unlikely to occur in an otherwise healthy heart.
F **e** May be treated successfully with intravenous digoxin.

---

59 **Bronchospasm during anaesthesia may be treated with**

T **a** Aminophylline.
T **b** Salbutamol.
T **c** Ether.

F **d** Metoprolol.
T **e** Sodium cromoglycate.

(Ch. 36, A & S)

a True This is the result of inhaling gaseous products of combustion. Carbon monoxide has a high affinity for haemoglobin. High concentrations in burned patients lead to tissue hypoxia.

b False The acute response to stress leads to hyperventilation.

c True In children i.v. fluids are required if the burn area is > 10%.

d False 50% of i.v. fluid replacement should be given as albumin solution.

e False Suxamethonium is hazardous in the later period between approximately 1 week and 3 months.

(Ch. 37, A & S)

a True It acts by competing for acetylcholine receptor sites at the autonomic ganglia.

b True It is a sympathetic and parasympathetic ganglion blocker.

c False Cycloplegia occurs after administration of hexamethonium.

d False

e False It undergoes metabolism in the liver.

(Ch. 16, A & S)

a False Critical temperature is that temperature above which it is not possible to liquefy a gas even with infinite pressure.

b False See above.

c False See above.

d True The gas in equilibrium with its liquid in this case is strictly termed a vapour.

e True

(Ch. 7, D)

a True The rate may be slowed by carotid sinus massage.

b True This may indicate the need for treatment with a beta-blocker.

c True See above.

d True In contrast to paroxysmal atrial tachycardia without A–V block.

e True Digoxin may be used to control the ventricular rate; however, A–V block may occur as a toxic effect of digoxin therapy.

(Ch. 23, A & S)

a True This is given slowly i.v. in a dose of 250–500 mg.

b True This is a specific $beta_2$-adrenoceptor agonist. *(Ch. 13, A & S)*

c True Ether has sympathomimetic actions and has been used to treat bronchospasm during anaesthesia. *(Ch. 9, A & S)*

d False This is a selective $beta_1$-blocker. *(Ch. 13, A & S)*

e False Sodium cromoglycate may be used therapeutically for prophylaxis against histamine release, but not for direct treatment.

60   The Magill attachment

a   Is an example of a Mapleson E system.

b   Is functionally similar to the Lack system.

c   Is economical in terms of fresh gas flow rate when used for IPPV.

d   For spontaneous respiration needs a FGF rate of > 70 ml/kg.

e   Can be used for children > 25 kg.

(Ch. 17, Appx. VII, A & S)

a False It is described by Mapleson as an 'A' system – the Mapleson 'E' system is represented by the Ayre's 'T' piece.

b True The Lack system is a coaxial version of the Magill attachment, but is not as efficient.

c False High fresh gas flow rates are required to obviate carbon dioxide rebreathing when this system is used for IPPV.

d True This figure is derived from the expected alveolar minute ventilation.

e True This is the lower limit of weight for the use of this system.
(Appx. 7, A & S)

6. Examination 2

---

1   **Plasma cholinesterase**

a   Is manufactured in the liver.

b   Cleaves the amide bond of suxamethonium.

c   Is absent in homozygotes for atypical cholinesterase.

d   When absent, is treated with fresh frozen plasma (FFP).

e   Is reduced in concentration by haemofiltration.

---

2   **The following statements are correct**

a   Acidosis associated with diabetic coma is caused by vomiting.

b   Acidosis associated with diarrhoea is caused by loss of base.

c   Acidosis during renal failure is caused by decreased sodium excretion.

d   Metabolic alkalosis may be reversed with i.v. saline.

e   When blood is taken from a patient at 32°C, the measured Pa_{CO_2} is higher when the sample is analysed at 37°C.

(Ch. 12, A & S)

a **True** This is one of the proteins synthesised by the liver.

b **False** There is no amide bond in suxamethonium, which comprises two molecules of acetylcholine joined by an ester link.

c **False** Patients homozygous for the atypical enzyme do not metabolise suxamethonium at a normal rate, but the concentration of plasma cholinesterase may be normal.

d **False** Treatment in such patients involves maintenance of ventilation and maintenance of anaesthesia while spontaneous metabolism occurs. FFP is not warranted in this situation.

e **False** Its concentration is reduced by plasmapheresis. Haemofiltration should have no effect.

---

a **False** It is caused by accumulation of ketone bodies as a result of increased lipolysis. *(Ch. 12, D)*

b **False** Alkalosis is more usual, secondary to hypokalaemia. Acidosis may be a manifestation of circulatory insufficiency. *(Ch. 22, A & S)*

c **False** Acidosis is caused by inability to excrete hydrogen ions. *(Ch. 11, D)*

d **True** This is the initial treatment of infants with pyloric stenosis, because the additional chloride ions permit renal excretion of bicarbonate. *(Ch. 5, D)*

e **True** Gas solubility is increased at lower temperatures. *(Ch. 16, A & S)*

3   Bupivacaine is

    a   Highly protein bound.

    b   Lipid-soluble.

    c   Causes methaemoglobinaemia.

    d   Suitable for continuous epidural anaesthesia.

    e   Highly cardiotoxic.

4   The following are true of gas cylinders

    a   Oxygen is supplied in cylinders at a pressure of 120 lb/in^2.

    b   Nitrous oxide is supplied at a pressure of 44 lb/in^2.

    c   Full nitrous oxide cylinders contain only liquid nitrogen.

    d   Nitrous oxide cylinders should not be stored below −7°C.

    e   Helium cylinders are coloured pink.

5   Enchanced neuromuscular blockade occurs with the following combinations

    a   Suxamethonium and neostigmine.

    b   D-tubocurarine and ecothiopate.

    c   Alcuronium and tobramycin.

    d   Gallamine and atropine.

    e   Vecuronium and isoflurane.

(Ch. 15, A & S)

a True 95% of bupivacaine in blood is bound to protein.
b True In common with all local anaesthetic agents, bupivacaine is lipid soluble.
c False Bupivacaine has not been associated with methaemoglobinaemia – this complication is usually ascribed to prilocaine.
d True Bupivacaine is the agent of choice for continuous epidural anaesthesia.
e True Bupivacaine is amongst the most cardiotoxic of all the local anaesthetic agents. *(Ch. 15, BNF)*

(Ch. 17, A & S)

a False The usual pressure in a full oxygen cylinder is 13.7 MPa – approximately 2000 lb/in^2.
b False Nitrous oxide cylinders are supplied usually with a pressure of 44 bar (750 lb/in^2).
c False Nitrous oxide cylinders contain liquid nitrous oxide!
d True All gas cylinders for medical use should be stored in a warm dry place and not subjected to extremes of temperature. $-7°C$ is the pseudocritical temperature for Entonox.
e False Helium cylinders are brown.

(Ch. 12, A & S)

a True One of the characteristics of a depolarising block is that an anticholinesterase (such as neostigmine) may make the block more intense.
b False Ecothiopate depresses plasma cholinesterase. There is no interaction with a nondepolarising drug, such as curare.
c True The intraperitoneal administration of aminoglycoside antibiotics may prolong the effect of nondepolarising neuromuscular blockers.
d False The anti-muscarinic actions of atropine have no influence on neuromuscular blocking drugs.
e True The use of inhalational anaesthetics, especially isoflurane and enflurane, prolongs the neuromuscular blockade induced by non-depolarising agents.

6   The following are more soluble in water than in blood

    a   Ether.

    b   Nitrous oxide.

    c   Halothane.

    d   Methoxyflurane.

    e   Isoflurane.

7   During one-lung ventilation

    a   A double-lumen bronchial tube is required.

    b   Increased intrapulmonary shunting results in decreased Pa_{O_2}.
    c   Increased intrapulmonary shunting results in decreased Sa_{O_2}.
    d   Increased intrapulmonary shunting results in increased Pa_{CO_2}.

    e   An $F_{I_{O_2}}$ of 0.6 or greater is necessary.

8   In a patient who has received alpha-adrenoceptor blockers, the following would be expected

    a   Cold skin.
    b   Miosis.

    c   Decreased arterial pressure.
    d   Orthostatic hypotension.

    e   Bradycardia.

9   A 2.5% solution of thiopentone injected intra-arterially causes fewer problems than a 5% solution because

    a   Less microcrystals and micro-aggregates are formed.

    b   It is less alkaline.
    c   It is isotonic, whereas the 5% solution is hypertonic.
    d   The pH of the 2.5% solution is neutral.
    e   It is more easily dispersed in the arterial blood.

(Appx. II, A & S)

a **True** The water/gas solubility coefficient of ether is 13, and its blood/gas coefficient is 12.
b **False** Water/gas solubility coefficient 0.44; blood/gas solubility coefficient 0.47.
c **False** Water/gas solubility coefficient 0.8; blood/gas solubility coefficient 2.5.
d **False** Water/gas solubility coefficient 4.5; blood/gas solubility coefficient 13.
e **False** Water/gas solubility coefficient 0.62; blood/gas solubility coefficient 1.4.

(Ch. 39, A & S)

a **True** In theory, single-lumen tubes may be employed, but a double-lumen tube is the commonest type used for this purpose.
b **True** Shunting occurs through the non-ventilated lung.
c **True** Decreased saturation accompanies the decrease in Pa_{O_2}.
d **False** Carbon dioxide excretion is relatively unaffected by one-lung ventilation.
e **False** Inspired oxygen concentration in excess of 60% does not increase oxygen delivery and may negate the useful effect of hypoxic pulmonary vasoconstriction.

(Ch. 13, A & S)

a **False** Alpha-adrenoceptor blockade results in peripheral vasodilatation.
b **True** The sympathetic supply to the pupil via alpha-adrenoceptors produces pupillary dilation.
c **True** Peripheral vasoconstrictor tone is reduced with alpha-blockade.
d **True** The normal physiological response on assuming the upright posture is peripheral vasoconstriction mediated via alpha-adrenoceptors.
e **False** The chronotropic supply to the heart is mediated via beta-adrenoceptors.

(Ch. 10, A & S)

a **True** Crystal formation is thought to be related to the concentration of solution, and thus the 2.5% solution is safer.
b **False** The pH of a solution (whether 2.5% or 5%) of thiopentone is 10.5.
c **False** The tonicity of the fluid is not the limiting factor in this case.
d **False** See **b** above.
e **False** See **a** above.

10   An increase in minute volume may be caused by

   a   Increased CSF H$^+$ concentration.

   b Pa_{O_2} of 8 kPa.

   c   A chronic anaemia of Hb 5 g/dl.

   d   Intravenous adrenaline.

   e   Breathing 0.03% CO_2 in air.

11   The following are complications of gallstones

   a   Pancreatitis.

   b   Cholangitis.

   c   Hiatus hernia.

   d   Intestinal obstruction.

   e   Carcinoma of the gall bladder.

12   Rate of gastric emptying is diminished by the following drugs in therapeutic dosage

   a   Atropine.

   b   Morphine.

   c   Apomorphine.

   d   Codeine.

   e   Neostigmine.

(Ch. 2, A & S)

a True This is the normal physiological mechanism whereby central chemoreceptor stimulation results in an increase in minute volume.

b False Peripheral hypoxic stimulation increases minute volume only if Pa_{O_2} is less than 8 kPa in the presence of a normal Pa_{CO_2}.

c False In chronic anaemia, there is a compensatory increase in 2, 3-DPG concentration in the red cell, and tissue oxygenation is impaired less than in acute anaemia. *(Ch. 7, A & S)*

d True Exogenous catecholamine stimulation of the cardiovascular and respiratory systems occurs.

e False 0.03% CO_2 is the normal value for concentration of carbon dioxide in air.

(Ch. 10, D)

a True There is a frequent association between disease of the biliary tract and pancreatitis. *(Ch. 9, D)*

b True

c False This is not a complication of cholelithiasis, although the two conditions may co-exist.

d True A large gallstone may reach the intestinal tract and cause obstruction, usually at the terminal ileum.

e False Carcinoma of the gall bladder is very uncommon, whereas gallstones are present in 15–20% of the adult population, the frequency being greater than 40% in those over 60 years of age.

(Ch. 19, Ch 11, A & S)

a True Atropine is an anticholinergic and therefore inhibits gastrointestinal motility.

b True This has a profound inhibitory effect upon the rate of gastric emptying; this is not antagonised by metoclopramide.

c False This induces vomiting and therefore increases the rate of gastric emptying!

d True This inhibits gastrointestinal motility.

e False This does not delay gastric emptying.

13 If surgery is required in a patient who has suffered myocardial infarction

a There is at least a tenfold increase in the risk of reinfarction if surgery occurs within 3–6 months of a previous myocardial infarction.

b Hypotension is desirable during anaesthesia to reduce cardiac work.

c No opioid premedication should be given.

d Tracheal intubation should be undertaken only during a light plane of anaesthesia.

e Halothane should be avoided.

14 Irrigation of the bladder during surgery for TURP may result in

a Hyponatraemia.

b Haemodilution.

c Haemolysis.

d Hyperkalaemia.

e Hypercalcaemia.

15 Tolerance to opioids

a Is always associated with dependence.

b Results in tolerance to barbiturates.

c Is caused by enzyme induction.

d Is not agonist-specific.

e Is increased commonly in alcoholics.

16 In the infant undergoing general anaesthesia

a The larynx is placed higher in the neck than in the adult.

b The use of the Macintosh laryngoscope is recommended.

c The tracheal tube should be (age/4 + 4.5) mm internal diameter.

d Preformed tracheal tubes avoid endobronchial intubation.

e A praecordial stethoscope provides an index of cardiac output.

(Ch. 41, A & S)

a True Within 3–6 months of myocardial infarction, the risk of reinfarction is approximately 16%.

b False Maintenance of normotension is desirable during anaesthesia; hypotension reduces coronary blood flow if the arteries are stenosed.

c False Premedication should be sufficient to allay anxiety.

d False Deep anaesthesia is required to obtund the increases in heart rate and arterial pressure associated with tracheal intubation.

e False Small concentrations of halothane may be beneficial by depressing myocardial oxygen consumption.

(Ch. 27, A & S)

a True Dilutional hyponatraemia may occur because of absorption of irrigation fluid into venous sinuses.

b True Haemodilution and reduction in haematocrit may indicate absorption of large volumes of fluid.

c False Haemolysis is not a feature of dilutional hyponatraemia.

d False Absorption of irrigating solution does not cause an increase in serum potassium concentration.

e False Calcium is not a constituent of bladder irrigating solutions.

(Ch. 16, D; Ch. 4, BNF)

a False Dependence and tolerance are separate entities. Acute tolerance may occur without dependence, but tolerance may occur also as a consequence of dependence.

b False Cross-tolerance does not occur, but enzyme inducers, e.g. ethyl alcohol, may result in tolerance to intravenous barbiturates.

c False Tolerance may develop to all opioids, but this is not related to enzyme induction.

d True Cross-tolerance may occur with all opioid analgesics.

e False Classically, alcoholics demonstrate tolerance to barbiturate drugs.

(Ch. 34, A & S)

a True The larynx is at C3–4 compared with C5–6 in the adult.

b False Laryngoscopy is easier with a straight-bladed laryngoscope.

c False The size required is: age/4 + 4 mm.

d False Preformed tubes of fixed length may result in bronchial intubation.

e True In the infant, the intensity of sound varies with the stroke volume.

17 **Infrared gas analysis is a suitable technique for measurement of clinical concentrations of**

F a Oxygen.

T b Nitrous oxide.

T c Carbon dioxide.

F d Helium.   *inert gas   no absorp*

X e Ethyl alcohol.   *Spech in infrare.*

T   *infrared vapour analyse*

18 **Increased serum urea concentration after a large haematemesis may be caused by**

T a Dehydration.

F b Potassium loss.   *net acidosis*

F c Metabolic acidosis.   *↑Hᵗ*

T d Depressed renal function.

T e Increased protein catabolism in the gut.

19 **Ethanol causes**

T a Enzyme induction in the liver.

T b Vasodilatation in skin.

F c Antagonism of respiratory depression caused by barbiturates.

T d Direct liver cell damage.

T e Peripheral neuropathy.   *— No*
          B₁₂

20 **Ventricular ectopic beats**

F a May be differentiated from atrial fibrillation by inspection of the peripheral pulse.

T b May precipitate ventricular fibrillation after myocardial infarction.

T c Are associated with digoxin toxicity.

F d Are a good indicator of ischaemic heart disease.

F e May be treated with verapamil.

(Ch. 21, A & S)

a False Oxygen concentrations may be measured by paramagnetic, polarographic, or fuel cell analysis, and by mass spectrometry or chemically. Infrared analysis is not suitable.

b True Nitrous oxide has a peak absorption at 3.9 μm, which is well within the infrared spectrum. When infrared gas analysis is used to measure end-expired carbon dioxide, there may be interference from nitrous oxide.

c True This is the Luft principle described first in 1943, and employed routinely in capnography.

d False Helium is an inert gas and does not have a suitable absorption spectrum in the infrared range.

e True An infrared vapour analyser can be used to measure expired ethyl alcohol concentration.

(Ch. 9, D)

a True Dehydration results from movement of interstitial fluid into the circulation to replace the lost blood.

b False This is not a feature of this condition.

c False The serum urea concentration is not influenced by acid-base abnormalities.

d True Blood loss and hypotension may result in renal failure.

e True For this reason, antibiotics are frequently administered to patients with gastrointestinal bleeding.

(Ch. 16, D)

a True Microsomal enzyme induction may occur with chronic alcohol abuse.

b True Ethanol is a potent peripheral vasodilator.

c False Ethanol is a CNS depressant and does not reverse depression caused by other CNS depressants.

d False Unlike chloroform, ethanol does not cause direct liver cell damage.

e True This may occur in the alcoholic because of nutritional deficiency.
(Ch. 15, D)

(Ch. 7, D)

a False An ECG is required for accurate diagnosis.

b True This is more likely if an ectopic beat coincides with the T wave of the previous complex.

c True Bigeminy is common.

d False Ventricular ectopic beats may occur in normal individuals.

e False The main indication for verapamil is supraventricular tachycardia.

21 **Intermittent positive pressure ventilation (IPPV) in the anaesthetised patient results in:**

a Decreased functional residual capacity (FRC).

b Increased lung compliance.

c Increased intrapleural pressure.

d Decreased cardiac output in hypovolaemia.

e Increased right atrial pressure.

the pressure

---

22 **The risk of fire in the operating room may be reduced by**

a Connecting trolleys by a high resistance to the floor.

b Avoiding battery operated equipment whenever possible.

c The use of an isolation transformer.

d Use of footwear with a resistance of 10 000 ohms.

e Siting electrical sockets higher than 1.5 m above the floor.

---

23 **Fresh frozen plasma**

a Must be crossmatched.

b May be used to treat DIC.

c Is used during massive blood transfusion.

d Is indicated in the treatment of burns.

e Is indicated in the treatment of renal failure.

just giving Ab → not sensitised then

a True FRC is reduced during anaesthesia to a similar extent by either IPPV or spontaneous ventilation.

b False Lung compliance remains unchanged, or may decrease if a low tidal volume is employed.

c True IPPV increases intrapleural pressure during inspiration.

d True The increased intrapulmonary and intrathoracic pressures reduce venous return to the heart especially in the hypovolaemic patient, and results in a decreased cardiac output. *(Ch. 3, A & S)*

e True Increased intrathoracic pressure is transmitted to the great vessels and right atrium.

a True Trolleys are connected to the floor by a high resistance; this prevents the accumulation of static electrical charges whilst maintaining electrical isolation for mains voltages (240 V r.m.s.).

b False Such equipment is recommended because the low voltage employed reduces the risk of sparks.

c True An isolation transformer reduces the risk of electrocution, but not of spark formation.

d False Footwear designed for use in the operating theatre should have a resistance of greater than 1 Mohm.

e True Most inflammable vapours are heavier than air.

a False Rhesus compatibility is not required but it must be ABO compatible.

b True FFP is rich in heat-labile coagulation factors. *(Appx. VIII, A & S)*

c True Massive blood transfusion may lead to dilutional coagulopathy. This is treated with FFP, platelets, and, sometimes, factor VIII concentrate. *(Ch. 36, A & S)*

d True Burns produce a rapid loss of plasma protein (including the plasma coagulation factors which are present in fresh frozen plasma). *(Ch. 36, A & S)*

e False There is no specific indication for using fresh frozen plasma in renal failure.

24   Suxamethonium

a   Must be stored below 4°C.

b   Causes a reduction in intracellular potassium concentration.

c   Increases intraocular pressure because of an increase in venous pressure.

d   Its action is prolonged in liver failure.

e   Is contraindicated in severe burns.

25   Which of the following measurements are satisfactory for assessing adequate recovery of neuromuscular function

a   Minute volume.

b   Generation of an inspiratory pressure of –60 cm H_2O.

c   Head lift sustained for 5 seconds.

d   Tidal volume.

e   Respiratory rate.

26   An obese patient is more likely to demonstrate

a   Difficulty on tracheal intubation.

b   Hypoxaemia.

c   Abnormal sensitivity to muscle relaxants.

d   Abnormal sensitivity to thiopentone.

e   Hypertension.

27   The Bain system

a   Cannot be sterilised.

b   Is a variant of the Mapleson A breathing system.

c   Is dangerous if the inner tube becomes disconnected at the patient end.

d   Has tubing of >1 m in length.

e   Should be used with a fresh gas flow equal to minute volume during spontaneous ventilation.

(Ch. 12, A & S)

a **True**   Some deterioration occurs if it is stored above this temperature.
b **True**   This is associated with an increase in extracellular potassium concentration. *(Ch. 23, A & S)*
c **True**   The increase in intra-ocular pressure caused by suxamethonium is caused partly by an increase in venous pressure. Contraction of the tonic fibres of extra-ocular muscles is also contributory.
d **True**   Plasma cholinesterase concentration is decreased in the presence of hepatic failure.
e **True**   Hyperkalaemia is particularly marked in patients with severe burns, extensive muscle damage, recently paraplegic patients, and patients with peripheral neuropathies. *(Ch. 23, A & S)*

(Ch. 24, A & S)

a **False**   This is not a reliable measure of recovery, as normal values may be achieved during partial paralysis.
b **True**
c **True**   This indicates absence of fade.
d **False**   Although this may be adequate whilst neuromuscular recovery is incomplete, it indicates that recovery is occurring.
e **False**   Respiratory rate depends upon respiratory drive, and is independent of neuromuscular transmission.

(Ch. 41, A & S)

a **True**   In the morbidly obese, direct laryngoscopy may be difficult to perform. *(Ch. 23, A & S)*
b **True**   This occurs because of a decrease in FRC and increase in airway closure.
c **False**   Abnormal sensitivity does not exist. However, if drugs are given on a body weight basis, overdosage may result.
d **False**   See above.
e **True**   But care should be taken not to overestimate arterial pressure because an inappropriately small sphygmomanometer cuff is used.

(Ch. 17, A & S)

a **False**   The components of the Bain system may be sterilised by heat.
b **False**   It is a variant of the Mapleson D system.
c **False**   Disconnection at the machine end is dangerous as it results in rebreathing of carbon dioxide.
d **True**   The volume of the tubing must be greater than the patient's tidal volume. One metre of 22 mm tubing has a volume of about 600 ml.
e **False**   Fresh gas flow rate should be 2–3 times the minute volume to prevent rebreathing during spontaneous ventilation. *(Appx. VII, A & S)*

28 **Reduction in blood glucose concentration is caused by**

a Isoprenaline.

b Phenformin.

c Tolbutamide.

d Hydrocortisone.

e Alpha-adrenergic blocking agents.

29 **A serum potassium concentration of 2.5 mmol/litre and serum bicarbonate concentration of 15 mmol/litre are compatible with**

a Treatment of diabetic ketoacidosis with insulin alone.

b Primary hyperaldosteronism.

c Large volume of blood transfusion.

d Pyloric stenosis.

e Ventilatory failure in chronic bronchitis.

30 **Dilatation of the cervix may result in**

a Laryngospasm.

b Tachycardia.

c Bradycardia.

d Postoperative shivering.

e Intense bleeding.

31 **In day case anaesthesia**

a Tracheal intubation is contraindicated.

b Ketamine is a useful agent.

c After circumcision under caudal analgesia, micturition is often delayed.

d Patients may be permitted to drive or operate machinery after 12 hours.

e Thiopentone is not contraindicated for induction.

a False Isoprenaline is a beta-adrenergic agonist with a predominant action on beta$_1$-intracardiac receptors. *(Ch. 2, BNF)*

b True Phenformin is a biguanide oral hypoglycaemic agent with a strong propensity to cause lactic acidosis. Metformin is the only biguanide now available. *(Ch. 12, D; Ch. 6, BNF)*

c True Tolbutamide is a sulphonylurea hypoglycaemic agent with a short duration of action. *(Ch. 6, BNF)*

d False Steroids tend to promote glycogenolysis and gluconeogenesis.

e False Alpha-adrenoceptor blockers act on peripheral receptors and have no pancreatic action. *(Ch. 5, A & S)*

(Ch. 22, A & S; Ch. 5, D)

a True But metabolic acidosis may result in hyperkalaemia.

b False Metabolic alkalosis usually accompanies potassium depletion. *(Ch. 12, D)*

c False This may produce transient hyperkalaemia.

d False This usually causes alkalosis. *(Ch. 9, D)*

e False This may result in compensated respiratory acidosis: the serum bicarbonate concentration would be elevated. *(Ch. 8, D)*

(Ch. 27, A & S)

a True This may occur under light anaesthesia.

b False Bradycardia is the usual response.

c True Because of insufficient depth of anaesthesia.

d False This is associated with excessive use of volatile agents.

e False

(Ch. 31, A & S)

a False Provided that patients are supervised closely in the early postoperative period, there is no contraindication to tracheal intubation.

b False Dysphoric reactions, emergence phenomena and prolonged recovery preclude the usefulness of ketamine in this situation.

c True This is a common occurrence.

d False A minimum of 24 h is required.

e True Although slightly larger doses than normal may be necessary because premedication is usually omitted.

32 **Which of the following would lead you to postpone routine surgery or modify your anaesthetic technique**

a   Glycosuria on routine testing.

b   Haemoglobin concentration of 10.8 g/dl.

c   Bilirubinaemia.

d   White cell count of 8.0×10^9/litre.

e   Serum potassium concentration of 2.5 mmol/litre.

33 **The following may be compressed together safely in a cylinder**

a   Helium and oxygen.

b   Ethylene and oxygen.

c   Nitrous oxide and oxygen.

d   Carbon dioxide and oxygen.

e   Oxygen and acetylene.

34 **Lignocaine**

a   Is metabolised by plasma cholinesterases.

b   Has a longer duration of action than procaine.

c   Is destroyed by first pass metabolism after oral administration.

d   Can pass through mucous membranes.

e   Is an ester.

35 **Intrathecal morphine produces**

a   Nausea and vomiting.

b   Itching.

c   Respiratory depression.

d   Muscle weakness.

e   Urinary retention.

(Ch. 19, A & S)

a True This is not a reliable test of diabetes mellitus but would be an indication for further investigation.

b False A haemoglobin concentration of 10 g/dl is acceptable for routine surgery.

c True Bilirubinaemia is an indication for further investigation to elucidate its origin.

d False This is a normal white cell count.

e True This represents severe hypokalaemia and should be treated preoperatively.

(Ch. 17, A & S)

a True Helium (79%) and oxygen (21%) mixture is available in black cylinders with white and brown quartered shoulders at a pressure of 137 bar.

b False Ethylene is explosive. It is unwise to compress explosive gases with oxygen.

c True This is available as a 50% mixture as Entonox at a pressure of 137 bar.

d True Carbon dioxide and oxygen mixtures are available in black cylinders with white and grey quartered shoulders.

e False See **b**. Oxyacetylene welding equipment derives its supply from separate oxygen and acetylene cylinders.

(Ch. 15, A & S)

a False Lignocaine is an amide local anaesthetic agent. It was first synthesised in 1948.

b True Procaine is an ester-linked anaesthetic agent, metabolised by plasma cholinesterase.

c True There is significant metabolism of lignocaine in the liver. It also has a very short plasma half-life.

d True Care has to be taken that the toxic dose of 200 mg for an adult is not exceeded when lignocaine is applied to mucous membranes.

e False

(Ch. 11, A & S)

a True These are common side-effects.

b True Especially of the nose.

c True This may be severe and of late onset; it is recommended that after intrathecal administration of morphine, close supervision of the patient's respiration is maintained for *at least* 12 hours.

d False Muscle weakness is not associated with intrathecal morphine alone.

e True This is a distressing side-effect in 90% of males.

36   When anaesthetising a patient after head injury

F   a   Spontaneous ventilation is an acceptable technique.
T   b   Head flexion may increase intracranial pressure.
F   c   The patient should be well hydrated to ensure adequate cerebral blood flow.
T   d   Autoregulation may be impaired when mean arterial pressure (MAP) is < 80 mmHg.   60 ~ 160
    e   Opioids must be avoided.

---

37   The vapour concentration obtained from a Boyle's bottle containing liquid anaesthetic depends upon

F   a   Specific gravity of the liquid.
    b   The specific heat of the liquid.

T   c   Saturated vapour pressure of the liquid.
T   d   The latent heat of vaporisation of the liquid.

T   e   Gas flow rate.

---

38   Digoxin therapy in atrial fibrillation causes

T   a   Positive inotropic effect.
F   b   Positive chronotropic effect.
T   c   Increase in stroke volume.
    d   Increased refractory period of ventricular muscle.
    e   Delayed velocity of conduction in bundle of His.

---

39   Angina is a recognised feature of

T   a   Aortic stenosis.
T   b   Anaemia.
    c   Polyarthritis.
T   d   Hypothyroidism.
    e   Paroxysmal supraventricular tachycardia (SVT).

(Ch. 38, Ch. 32, A & S)

a False Increases in Pa_{CO_2} and ICP are likely to occur.
b True Head flexion may restrict the venous drainage from the cranium and cause an increase in ICP.
c True
d True The lower limit of autoregulation is normally 60 mmHg. However, autoregulation may be impaired at a higher arterial pressure in a patient with head injury.
e False There is no reason to avoid opioids provided that adequate ventilation is ensured.

(Ch. 16, A & S)

a False Specific gravity has no influence on vapour pressure.
b True Vaporisation is accompanied by a decrease in temperature. Specific heat determines rate of cooling and thus influences saturated vapour pressure.
c True
d True Latent heat of vaporisation determines the extent of cooling with evaporation. The temperature in turn influences the saturated vapour pressure.
e True The greater the gas flow, the greater is the total mass of vapour in the final gas mixture. However, at a given bypass setting, an increase in total gas flow rate decreases the delivered concentration.

(Ch. 7, D; Ch. 2, BNF)

a True But its main effect is to increase the degree of atrioventricular block and reduce ventricular rate.
b False The aim of digoxin therapy is to slow the ventricular rate.
c True As a result of the reduced ventricular rate, ventricular filling is improved and this may result in an increase in stroke volume.
d False The refractory period is shortened by digoxin therapy; this may result in ventricular tachycardia.
e True This is an important mechanism in controlling ventricular rate.

(Ch. 7, D)

a True
b True It may occur with severe anaemia (< 5 g/dl), especially in older patients. *(Ch. 13, D)*
c False Although aortic valvular disease may accompany polyarthritis, angina is not normally a feature.
d False In hypothyroidism the basal metabolic rate is depressed; angina is not a feature.
e True The increased oxygen demand produced by SVT may sometimes lead to angina.

40 The following arterial blood gas values: Pa_{O_2} 8 kPa; Pa_{CO_2} 4 kPa; pH 7.44; base excess −1 are compatible with

  a Alveolar hypoventilation.
  b Compensated metabolic alkalosis.
  c Lorrain-Smith effect.

  d Pulmonary atelectasis.
  e 48 h at an altitude of 3500 m.

41 Drugs used in the treatment of organophosphorus poisoning include

  a Neostigmine.

  b Pralidoxime.

  c Atropine.
  d Propranolol.
  e Chlorpromazine.

42 If helium is substituted for nitrogen in an air mixture the resultant gas

  a Is less dense.
  b Has a higher solubility in tissues.
  c Causes hypnosis.
  d Is more flammable.
  e Is used during upper airway obstruction.

43 Administration of quinidine may cause

  a Hypertension.
  b Increased refractory period of ventricular muscle.

  c Increased stroke volume.
  d Supraventricular tachycardia.
  e Circulatory arrest.

(Ch. 2, A & S)

a False Increased Pa_{CO_2} is characteristic of alveolar hypoventilation.
b False The base excess is positive in metabolic alkalosis. *(Ch. 22, A & S)*
c True The Lorrain-Smith effect describes pulmonary oxygen toxicity which may result subsequently in hypoxaemia.
d True This results in increased pulmonary shunt. *(Ch. 2, A & S)*.
e True Unacclimatised persons ascending to altitude hyperventilate.

(Ch. 17, D)

a False Organophosphorus compounds are cholinesterase inhibitors; neostigmine would enhance the poisoning.
b True Pralidoxime, a cholinesterase reactivator, has an action similar to that of atropine; treatment may need to be repeated every 30 min as necessary.
c True See **a.**
d False Propranolol is a beta-adrenergic blocker.
e False Chlorpromazine does not possess anticholinergic properties.

(Ch. 16, A & S)

a True The density of the mixture of helium is about one-third that of air.
b False Helium is less soluble than nitrogen.
c False Helium is an inert gas and is not narcotic.
d False Helium is not flammable.
e True As a result of its lower density, helium/oxygen flows at a greater rate than air during turbulence.

(Ch. 7, D; Ch. 2, BNF)

a False Quinidine is a myocardial depressant and may cause hypotension.
b False Ventricular conduction is slowed, because of slowing of the sodium current across the cell membrane.
c False Quinidine is a myocardial depressant.
d False This is one of the indications for quinidine therapy.
e True As a result of a combination of myocardial and conducting system depression.

44 **The volume of fluid flowing in a laminar fashion through a tube is directly proportional to**

   a The density of the fluid.

   b The length of the tube.
   c The pressure difference across the tube.
   d The fourth power of the radius of the tube.
   e The viscosity of the fluid.

---

45 **Which of the following are true of the soda lime used in a circle system?**

   a It should fill at least half of the canister.

   b It requires water for CO_2 to be absorbed.
   c It may absorb up to 20% of its weight of CO_2.
   d It consists mainly of calcium carbonate.
   e Its indicator changes from white to pink with use.

---

46 **Ketamine should be avoided**

   a In the presence of increased arterial pressure.

   b In pregnancy.
   c In shock.

   d In the asthmatic.

   e In the presence of facial burns.

---

47 **Pulse pressure increases with**

   a Moderate increase in total peripheral resistance.
   b Increased stroke volume.

   c Atherosclerosis.

   d Decreased blood viscosity.

   e Moderate hypercapnia.